THE TOBACCO ATLAS

SIXTH EDITION

 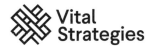

www.tobaccoatlas.org

The Tobacco Atlas
Sixth Edition
A Companion to the TobaccoAtlas.org Website

Jeffrey Drope, PhD and Neil W. Schluger, MD, Editors

Published by the American Cancer Society, Inc.
250 Williams Street
Atlanta, Georgia 30303 USA
www.cancer.org

Suggested citation:
Drope J, Schluger N, Cahn Z, Drope J, Hamill S, Islami F, Liber A, Nargis N, Stoklosa M.
2018. The Tobacco Atlas. Atlanta: American Cancer Society and Vital Strategies.

ISBN: 978-1-60443-257-2
Publisher's Cataloging-in-Publication Data

Names: Drope, Jeffrey, author. | Schluger, Neil W., 1959- author. | Zachary Cahn, author.
| Jacqui Drope, author. | Stephen Hamill, author. | Farhad Islami, author. | Alex Liber,
author. | Nigar Nargis, author. | Michal Stoklosa, author.
Title: The tobacco atlas / Jeffrey Drope and Neil W. Schluger, editors, with Zachary
Cahn, Jacqui Drope, Stephen Hamill, Farhad Islami, Alex Liber, Nigar Nargis and Michal
Stoklosa.
Description: Sixth edition. | American Cancer Society, Inc. and Vital Strategies. | Atlanta
[Georgia] : 2018. | Includes index.
Identifiers: LCCN pending. | ISBN: 978-1-60443-257-2 (pbk. : alk. paper)
Subjects: 1. Tobacco use—Maps. 2. Tobacco use—Statistics—Maps. 3. Tobacco
industry—Maps. 4. Medical geography—Maps.
Classification: LCC pending | DDC 362.29'60223—dc23

Managing Editor: John M. Daniel
Contributing Editor: Johnny J. Hsu

Printed by RR Donnelley
Printed in China

Design: Radish Lab, www.radishlab.com
304 Boerum St, Suite 42
Brooklyn, NY 11206

Illustration: Daniel Stolle, danielstolle.com

TABLE OF CONTENTS

FOREWORD

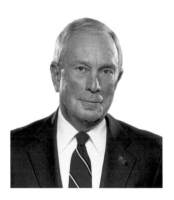

Tobacco will kill one billion (1,000,000,000) people this century, if we do nothing. It is the world's leading preventable killer, driving an epidemic of cancer, heart disease, stroke, chronic lung disease and other non-communicable diseases. But the good news is: we know the most effective strategies for stopping it. The challenge we face is persuading more leaders to embrace them— and empowering those leaders to implement them.

For almost two decades *The Tobacco Atlas* has been turning the most up-to-date global data into compelling and easy-to-understand graphics. With a changing landscape of products, determined industry opposition, and promising new tobacco control strategies, arming advocates with accurate and persuasive data has never been more important.

Governments should act now to implement WHO's MPOWER policies and other proven interventions to create a significantly healthier future. I hope, in the pages of this sixth edition of *The Tobacco Atlas*, public health advocates find new tools for spurring action.

MICHAEL R. BLOOMBERG
World Health Organization Global Ambassador for Non-Communicable Disease
Bloomberg Philanthropies

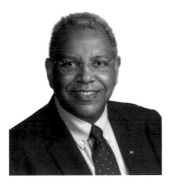

OTIS W. BRAWLEY
Chief Medical Officer,
American Cancer Society

The sixth edition of *The Tobacco Atlas* celebrates recent achievements in tobacco control, illuminates the myriad harms of tobacco use, and offers a set of proven tools to advance a tobacco-free world. The data depict a sobering look at the daunting magnitude of the epidemic, but also show considerable progress in places where governments take up solutions that are proven to work. For the first time, more than two billion people are protected by at least one WHO MPOWER measure, but very few countries have taken up every measure. Our life-saving opportunity lies in that gap.

In the last few years, tobacco control has been rightly seen as a crucial element of the movement for human development. In addition to saving millions of lives, tobacco control policies can improve livelihoods and drive enormous economic benefits by preventing the vast economic costs of tobacco-related diseases. Recent estimates suggest that these costs are close to a staggering two percent of the entire world's gross domestic product. Imagine if we could reallocate these lost resources to initiatives that increase prosperity, such as improved health and education.

We note that the ultimate path to improved tobacco control is political will. We must foster political will and all it portends for saving lives by prioritizing efforts that lead to action. The data are clear that measures like raising taxes and enacting 100% smoke-free air laws indisputably work, but too many governments have not yet committed to adopting them. For those governments that think they lack adequate resources to pursue effective strategies, *The Tobacco Atlas* demonstrates a significant return on investment. And for any governments that still listen to the arguments of the tobacco industry, which has long proven its indifference to health and life, *The Tobacco Atlas* systematically debunks its myths and displays its depravity.

One of the prominent themes of the *Atlas* is cooperation. We are proud that our two organizations have worked together for almost two decades to engender a healthier world. We urge governments, advocates, organizations and people who care about these issues to stand with us and shoulder-to-shoulder with the many who seek to reduce this man-made epidemic in pursuit of a healthier planet.

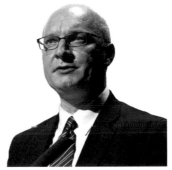

JOSÉ LUIS CASTRO
Executive Director, The Union
President and CEO, Vital Strategies

ABOUT THE TOBACCO ATLAS AUTHORS

Editor-Authors

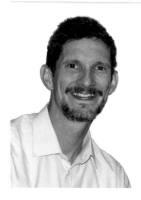

JEFFREY DROPE, PhD, is Vice President, Economic and Health Policy Research at the American Cancer Society. He is also Professor in Residence of Global Public Health at Marquette University. His research and capacity-building efforts focus principally on the nexus of risk factors for cancer (e.g., tobacco use, poor nutrition and physical inactivity) and economic policy (e.g., taxation, trade and investment).

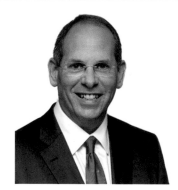

NEIL W. SCHLUGER, MD, is Senior Advisor for Science for Vital Strategies. He is also Professor of Medicine, Epidemiology and Environmental Health Science and Chief of the Division of Pulmonary, Allergy and Critical Care Medicine at Columbia University Medical Center in New York City.

Authors

ZACHARY CAHN, PhD, is Director, Economic and Health Policy Research at the American Cancer Society. His principal research focus is novel tobacco products.

JACQUI DROPE, MPH, is Managing Director of Global Cancer Prevention and Early Detection at the American Cancer Society. She leads programs at ACS that focus particularly on tobacco control and HPV vaccination across many low- and medium-HDI countries.

STEPHEN HAMILL is Vice President of Policy, Advocacy and Communication at Vital Strategies, a leading global public health organization. He supports governments in taking up cutting-edge policies like smoke-free indoor air laws or soda taxes, especially in low- and medium-HDI countries where prevention policies can save millions of lives.

FARHAD ISLAMI GOMESHTAPEH, MD, PhD, is Strategic Director, Cancer Surveillance Research in Surveillance and Health Services Research at the American Cancer Society. His work focuses on monitoring and describing trends in cancer occurrence in the United States and worldwide. He also conducts and collaborates on research on cancer disparities and cancer risk factors, particularly tobacco smoking.

ALEX LIBER, MSPH, is a Data Analyst in the Economic and Health Policy Research program at the American Cancer Society and a PhD Candidate at the University of Michigan's School of Public Health. Using multiple methodologies, his research focuses on issues in tobacco control policy and surveillance, including novel tobacco product regulation, tobacco pricing, and health insurance.

NIGAR NARGIS, PhD, is Director, Economic and Health Policy Research at the American Cancer Society. Her research and capacity-building efforts focus on issues related to tobacco taxation, tobacco affordability, tobacco use and poverty, and regressivity in some tobacco control policies.

MICHAL STOKLOSA, MA, is Senior Economist, Taxation & Health in the Economic and Health Policy Research program at the American Cancer Society, and a PhD Candidate in Economics at the University of Cape Town. He conducts research and trains policymakers and health advocates primarily in issues around tobacco taxation and illicit trade in tobacco products.

AUTHORS' PREFACE

It is with great passion and renewed urgency that we bring you the sixth edition of *The Tobacco Atlas*. In the 18 years since the first edition, there have been many positive changes in tobacco control: overall tobacco consumption has finally started to edge down, though this change is uneven across the globe. The WHO Framework Convention on Tobacco Control now has 181 parties and has truly become a vital blueprint for change.

Yet, tobacco use is increasing in some countries and within some sub-populations, particularly among the most vulnerable. We are launching this edition at the 2018 World Conference on Tobacco or Health in South Africa, on a continent that is a principal target of the tobacco industry's vigorous efforts to recruit new users. More broadly, the tobacco industry continues its nearly unfettered assault on public health. Some governments, despite having tools to improve tobacco control, continue to struggle to effect change, sometimes because of competing priorities, but in other cases simply due to a lack of effort.

In this edition, we first lay out the case for tobacco control. The death and destruction that follows in the wake of tobacco use is simply mind-boggling. But in the second half of the *Atlas*, we strive to emphasize the proven solutions that many in the public health community are actively utilizing with considerable success.

We are deeply grateful to our author/editor predecessors, both for atlas-style publications generally, and *The Tobacco Atlas* specifically. We particularly thank Judith Mackay and Michael Eriksen who were the early visionaries for this series—we hope that we have made them proud with this latest edition.

We are also extremely grateful to our organizations, the American Cancer Society and Vital Strategies, for their unwavering commitment to tobacco control and *The Tobacco Atlas*.

To save space in this print edition for content and to have more resources to pour into a dynamic website, the references are kept at www.tobaccoatlas.org (or www.ta6.org). We strongly encourage readers to visit our website for country fact sheets, considerable new content, frequent updates and comprehensive data, among other components.

In sum, we underscore here that while we continue to face a very serious challenge, we have the tools to make an enormous positive difference. We must persuade decision makers to make decisive, meaningful change, and where necessary, assist them to fight vigorously to implement these proven tools and enforce them. Finally, to achieve and sustain our shared goals, we are stronger working together— and we implore readers to seek out synergies with other forces to make sure tobacco control helps lead to a healthier, tobacco-free future.

Sincerely,

Jeff, Neil, Zach, Jacqui, Steve, Farhad, Alex, Nigar & Michal

PHOTO CREDITS

FIND MORE ON THE NEWLY EXPANDED AND UPDATED

www.tobaccoatlas.org

ACKNOWLEDGEMENTS

It takes many people to make a project like *The Tobacco Atlas* come together. At risk of excluding people who helped us along the way, we would like to acknowledge some very key actors.

First and foremost, Johnny Hsu at Vital Strategies and John Daniel at ACS might not have officially authored any chapters, but their roles were enormous and integral. Johnny anchored our design vision among many other tasks, while John went far beyond his official editorial responsibilities. The *Atlas* is a better product because of them.

At ACS, many folks played important roles. In terms of data and content preparation, we thank Samuel Asare, Martine Chaussard, Qing Li, and Nikisha Sisodiya. We couldn't have completed the project without the administrative and financial prowess of Nancy Inglis-Wesby and Shacquel Woodhouse, and the printing and publication expertise of Vanika Jordan. At Vital Strategies, we thank Christina Curell and Dane Svenson, but especially Tracey Johnston for her communications savvy among many other talents. Bob Land once again delivered an excellent index.

We are indebted to our talented design partners at Radish Lab. They were engaging, creative and hardworking every single day, including Hege Bryn (design), Kendall Holland (project management), and Eric Brelsford (data visualization).

We were a little skeptical about a publication anchored by illustrations, but Daniel Stolle has simply wowed us with his phenomenal vision and creativity. We are grateful for this new, wonderful twist to the *Atlas*.

We'd like to thank the leadership at both organizations. At ACS, our CEO Gary Reedy and CMO Otis Brawley, have strongly supported this publication. Similarly, at Vital Strategies, SVP Sandy Mullin has been a fervent supporter, as has the Union's Executive Director, José Luis Castro.

As we mention in the preface, we remain grateful to Michael Eriksen and Judith Mackay for their work on previous Atlases, and for their continuing support and collegiality.

Many colleagues generously helped along the way, including data, input, feedback, etc. on many chapters, including: Growing (Raphael Lencucha, Qing Li, and for the satellite images, Liora Sahar and Nick Faust); Manufacturing (Qing Li); Marketing (Lindsey Liber); Quitting (Martin Raw); Partnerships (Martine Chaussard and Mônica Andreis); Regulating Novel Products (Joanna Cohen, Ryan Kennedy, Robert Jackler, Cindy Chau and Divya Ramamurthi); Industry (Stella Bialous); and Countering the Industry (Deborah Arnott, Rob Cunningham and Holly Jarman).

For broader data needs, we thank the Institute for Health Metrics and Evaluation (IHME), particularly Emmanuela Gakidou, for generously permitting us to use many of their fantastic data to populate a number of maps and figures.

Any shortcomings, of course, are our own.

INTRODUCTION

By now, we know that tobacco kills more than half of those who regularly use it and has a two-trillion-dollar (purchasing power parity (PPP)) economic cost to society each year. Fortunately, the global community is making progress toward improving tobacco control. The efforts of governments, civil society and the international community, including through the WHO Framework Convention on Tobacco Control (FCTC), are having life-saving effects in many countries. Recently, overall global tobacco consumption has even decreased slightly. However, we continue to contend with the reality that many countries with young populations are experiencing growing prevalence as the tobacco industry's tactics continually undermine public health efforts.

This sixth edition of the *Tobacco Atlas* and its companion website— tobaccoatlas.org— bring readers and users an exciting and comprehensive guide to key tobacco control issues. It weaves together two related narratives: the bleak reality of the damage that tobacco causes even before it sprouts from the ground, and an optimistic examination of the evidence-based tools that we're using to address this reality, which could be further enhanced through more effective implementation.

We begin the narrative with cultivation of tobacco leaf, the foundation of every tobacco product. Here commences an enduring narrative of ill health and exploitation, in this case of the millions of mostly poor smallholder tobacco farmers. The tobacco industry turns the leaf into a variety of deadly tobacco products— most commonly cigarettes— and aggressively markets them, particularly to young people and other potentially vulnerable groups. In recent years, seeing opportunities in the lower prevalence among women and girls, and in many countries/regions low on the human development index (HDI), the industry has tailored its marketing efforts in this direction. It also continues to target many vulnerable populations in all countries. Accordingly, we explore global smoking and secondhand smoke prevalence followed by their results: adverse health effects, comorbidities, deaths from tobacco, and the broader costs to society.

The second half of the *Atlas* is more optimistic, focusing on the proven tools and strategies that we use to address the tobacco epidemic at almost every stage of the cycle of a tobacco product. These interventions include cessation efforts, marketing bans, smoke-free policies, tobacco taxes and mass media campaigns, among others. The market for tobacco products is also shifting in unpredictable ways. Some are optimistic that new non-combustible products that are potentially less harmful will diminish the market size of cigarettes and other combustible tobacco products. Others are understandably cautious about the uncertainty and any approach that involves tobacco companies, given their long history of deception and malfeasance.

The book can be read as a whole— a comprehensive narrative of the complete "cycle of tobacco"— or each chapter can be read on its own as a core component of this narrative. Importantly, we have developed a new, more dynamic companion website to 1) provide comprehensive, up-to-date data coverage; 2) address other important topics that we lack space to cover here (e.g., smokeless tobacco and water pipes); and 3) offer a place where we will regularly introduce timely and relevant new content. We hope the *Tobacco Atlas* will inspire you to action to improve tobacco control in your country, and will provide helpful guidance on the many tools to achieve these goals.

Fewer Smokers; Fewer Premature Deaths; $ Saved

If we meet the WHO's very tractable goal of a 30% relative reduction in each country by 2025, we would:

1. Have **173 million** fewer smokers
2. Prevent **38 million** premature deaths from smoking
3. Save **$16.9 trillion** (PPP) just from the former smokers becoming healthier and more productive.

Imagine if we set an even more ambitious target...

> **Instead of categorizing countries by income in the *Atlas*, we use the Human Development Index (HDI) because it moves beyond income to incorporate additional critical indicators such as health and education.**

FIND OUT MORE AT
www.tobaccoatlas.org/methods

CHAPTER KEY

 Inset   Web   Map

⊞ Wheel of Tobacco Regulation

Growing
Governments must help to improve supply and value chains for alternatives to tobacco leaf, and invest in farmers' education/re-training programs.

Manufacturing
Ban all tobacco additives, including flavorings.

Disposal
Get the tobacco industry to bear the cost of cleaning up the environmental devastation from the waste left by tobacco production and use.

Packaging and Labeling
Plain, standardized packaging of all tobacco products.

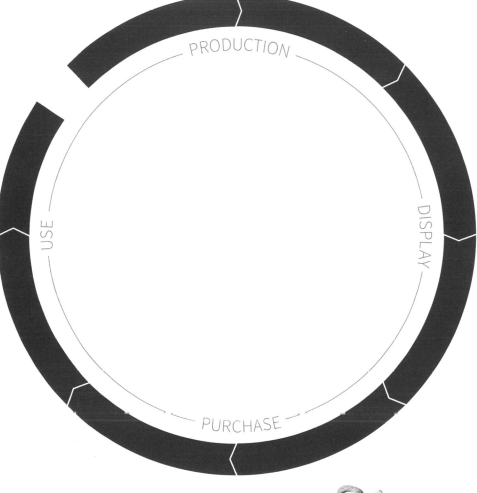

PRODUCTION

DISPLAY

USE

PURCHASE

Product Use
Policies should make all indoor, workplace and public outdoor spaces smoke-free, and find effective, new ways to keep smokers from smoking in their homes with non-smokers.

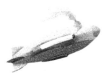

Marketing
Ban all direct and indirect forms of marketing, including advertising, promotion and sponsorship.

Point-of-Purchase
Eliminate all signs and even hints of tobacco product sales, including keeping them out of sight behind the counter.

Tax Policies
Implement higher excise taxes on all tobacco products and make certain that increases outpace inflation and income growth.

GROWING

Tobacco Leaf Production
by HDI, 1960-2014

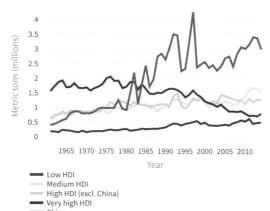

- Low HDI
- Medium HDI
- High HDI (excl. China)
- Very high HDI
- China

In the last few decades, China has come to dominate tobacco production, but notably production has dropped markedly in very high-HDI countries and increased everywhere else.

Smallholder Tobacco Farmer Profits

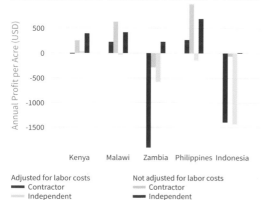

Kenya   Malawi   Zambia   Philippines   Indonesia

Adjusted for labor costs
- Contractor
- Independent

Not adjusted for labor costs
- Contractor
- Independent

All tobacco products start with a simple leaf. The cultivation of tobacco leaf, indigenous to the Americas, dates back at least eight millennia, and tobacco smoking for at least two. In the 15th century, Columbus helped shape the future of the tobacco industry as the first "importer" of tobacco into Europe. Within decades, tobacco had spread globally, including cultivation for commercial purposes. Mechanization of cigarette manufacturing in the 1880s helped grow the market for cigarettes dramatically, increasing demand for tobacco leaf.

While widespread cultivation of tobacco leaf has generated many challenges— including health hazards for farmers, environmental degradation and child labor issues—the most pressing systemic public health challenge is how the industry often uses tobacco farming to undermine tobacco control, arguing that tobacco control destroys the livelihoods of smallholder tobacco farmers. This specious argument—often perpetuated by governments' economic and/or agribusiness sectors—has resonated widely, undermining tobacco control efforts around the globe. Not coincidentally, tobacco farming has also shifted to some of the world's lowest-HDI countries, where governments are typically more economically and politically vulnerable.

Recent research across major tobacco-growing countries demonstrates that farming tobacco is not prosperous for most smallholder farmers. Many farmers—including many with contracts with oligopolistic leaf-buying companies—pay too much for inputs (e.g., fertilizer, pesticides, etc.),

receive very low prices for their leaf, and dedicate hundreds of hours to a mostly unprofitable economic pursuit. The opportunity costs of farming tobacco are high, with farmers missing out on human capital development and more lucrative economic opportunities.

So why do tobacco farmers grow tobacco? Many farmers report an assured market, even if prices are consistently low. Others report difficulty obtaining credit for other economic activities. For some, it is a way to generate cash in low-cash economies to pay for necessities like education and health care. Yet, the research demonstrates consistently that many tobacco farmers underestimate their costs and overestimate their returns.

Article 17 of the WHO FCTC compels Parties to promote viable alternative livelihoods for tobacco farmers. Few governments have made such efforts. There is no panacea for this transition; some countries have tried small programs to introduce new crops—e.g., bamboo in Kenya (with mixed results). Some farmers switch to and from tobacco, based on hopes for high leaf prices. The most successful larger-scale examples of change rely more on existing skills and experience. In Indonesia, former tobacco farmers are growing non-tobacco crops that they have always grown, and are making more money doing so. Governments can help by investing in supply and value chains, finding new markets for these other products, and divesting from any participation in tobacco cultivation. They can also re-invest vigorously in education and skills development, both agricultural and non-agricultural.

Tobacco Production by Volume
Metric tons, 2014

🌐 Explore more at ta6.org/growing

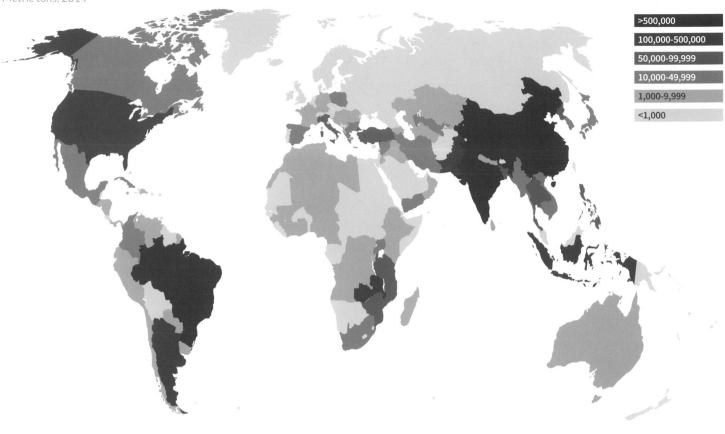

>500,000	
100,000-500,000	
50,000-99,999	
10,000-49,999	
1,000-9,999	
<1,000	

📊 Environmental Degradation from Tobacco Farming

Northern Region, Malawi
1992-2015 (2015 Landsat 8 image)

Western Tabora Region, Tanzania
1999-2017 (2017 Landsat 8 image)

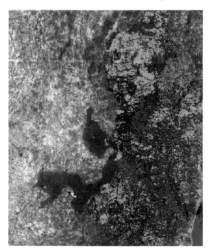

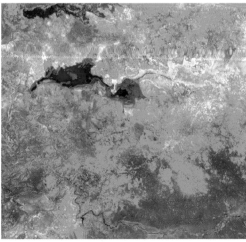

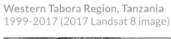 VEGETATION LOSS

In many countries, farmers clear forested land that is agriculturally marginal to grow tobacco—often by burning —and/or harvest wood for curing. Typically, the land is quickly abandoned and becomes unusable, often leading to desertification.

📊 Alternative Livelihoods
Indonesia Example

Crop (y-axis): Banana, Cashew and other Nuts, Cassava/Sweet Potato, Chili, Corn, Green Vegetables, Ground Nut, Mixed/Other, Paddy, Shallot

Region (x-axis): Upland Dry, Lowland Dry, Upland Wet, Lowland Wet

— Farmers who stopped growing tobacco
— Farmers still growing tobacco

Note: The circles indicate the size of sales of the crops.
Former tobacco farmers are growing more of most other local crops, making more money and spending less time in their fields than farmers continuing to grow tobacco.

CHAPTER 2
MANUFACTURING

Factory Consolidation

British American Tobacco closes factories, putting people out of work while handing over increasing gains to wealthy shareholders and executives

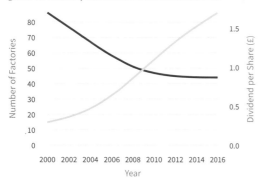

Factories
Share Dividend

Once raw tobacco leaf has been grown by a farmer and sold to a manufacturer, it must be processed into a desirable consumer product. To maximize profits, tobacco manufacturers want to make products that are as attractive and addictive as possible. The product standards governing this process of transformation aim to control tobacco products' characteristics and which kinds of tobacco products can be sold to consumers.

When these standards are written with public health in mind, tobacco products can be mandated to be less attractive and less addictive to users. Such strategies include bans on characterizing flavors, limits on nicotine content, and prohibitions against additives that quicken nicotine's absorption into the body. Additional policies include freezing the tobacco market by preventing the introduction of new brands, restricting a brand to a single presentation to prevent implicit suggestions of reduced harm in variants, and requiring the disclosure of ingredients to regulatory agencies and consumers.

Banning the addition of menthol, the most widely used flavor in tobacco products, has considerable potential to curb smoking. Research suggests that menthol in cigarettes may facilitate initiation and hinder quitting. Fortunately, laws banning the sale of menthol in tobacco products have passed in Brazil, Turkey, Ethiopia, the European Union, and five Canadian provinces.

While manufacturing standards that limit the appeal and addictiveness of products hold the promise of shrinking the tobacco market in the long run, there can be unintended consequences if such regulations do not carefully consider the broader tobacco product marketplace. For example, the market position of existing varieties of cigarettes became solidified when they were exempted from pre-market scrutiny under the United States' law extending the Food and Drug Administration's jurisdiction to cover tobacco products. Cigarette manufacturers were permitted to keep selling a deadly consumer product with only some restrictions, while barriers to the introduction of new potentially less harmful products were codified.

Meanwhile, the global tobacco industry has recently consolidated through privatization, acquisitions and mergers—now only 5 firms control 80% of the global cigarette market. These firms have automated and consolidated their own factories, steadily driving down the number of employees. Hence, now more than ever, when tobacco companies say that tobacco control policies threaten manufacturing jobs ⬛, we must remember that they are only in the business of maximizing their profits for shareholders, not protecting the well-being of their workers.

World's Largest-Producing Tobacco Product Factories
Where disease originates

🌐 Explore more at ta6.org/manufacturing

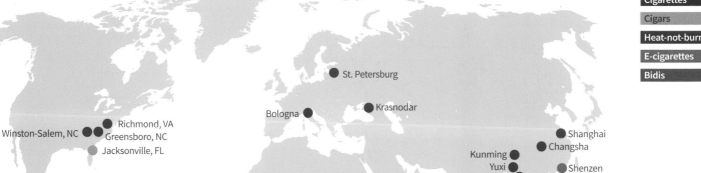

Legend:
- Cigarettes
- Cigars
- Heat-not-burn
- E-cigarettes
- Bidis

Map labels:
- St. Petersburg
- Bologna
- Krasnodar
- Shanghai
- Changsha
- Kunming
- Yuxi
- Shenzen
- Honghe
- Tamil Nadu
- Richmond, VA
- Winston-Salem, NC
- Greensboro, NC
- Jacksonville, FL

BAD PRACTICE

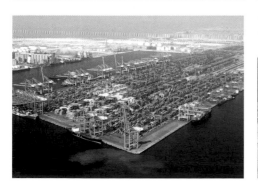

Free Trade Zone Cigarette Factories
One-third of illicit cigarette manufacturing facilities are located in free trade zones of the United Arab Emirates, Cyprus, and Russia, producing cigarettes that are smuggled into third-party countries, undermining tobacco control policy.

GOOD PRACTICE

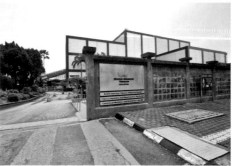

Resilience Facing Factory Closure
In 2016, British American Tobacco announced it would close its Petaling Jaya, Malaysia factory to consolidate manufacturing regionally, blaming high excise taxes on cigarettes. Malaysia did not bow to industry pressure to change its laws to try to save a factory.

CUTTING EDGE PRACTICE

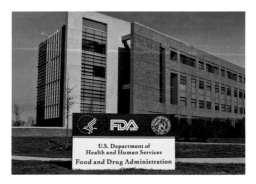

Mandatory De-Nicotinization
The United States FDA has begun proposing a rule mandating cigarette manufacturers lower nicotine levels to non-addictive or minimally addictive levels, potentially preventing millions from becoming addicted.

CHAPTER 3
MARKETING

Progress on Bans and Warnings

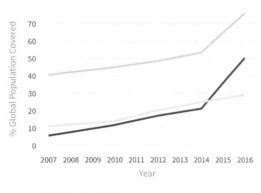

Percent of Global Population Covered by FCTC Marketing Policies (graphic health warnings (GHW) on packages, point-of-sale (POS) advertising ban, and internet marketing ban)

Legend:
- FCTC Compliant GHW
- POS Ad Ban
- Internet Ad Ban

Once a product rolls off the manufacturing line, it needs help to get to consumers. Tobacco companies must build the demand for products, particularly from new consumers. Marketing creates consumer demand, essentially inventing the reasons why a person would want to smoke a cigarette or use other tobacco products. Controlling the ability of the tobacco industry to spread favorable ideas about tobacco use is the essence of tobacco control efforts to regulate marketing. Closing off marketing channels to everyone has the primary benefit of shielding children from persuasive efforts that influence them to start smoking. While the tobacco industry always claims that their advertisements are not intended to appeal to children, they walk a fine line by aiming their marketing efforts to young adults, a group who children see as their closest peers and role models.

Sometimes, such as by marketing tobacco like candy, tobacco companies cross this line.

The tobacco industry has found creative ways to market its products, including through attractive packaging and so-called "corporate social responsibility" campaigns wherein they seek to present themselves as positive contributors to society. Regulating these myriad marketing strategies is a central tobacco control strategy. Essentially, wherever the tobacco industry tries to change the message about what their products represent away from disease and death, tobacco control attempts to change the conversation firmly back to the essential facts of tobacco use: disease and death.

Tobacco companies typically respond to marketing restrictions by reallocating resources to the remaining open channels. For example, when the government prohibits magazine and billboard advertising, the industry simply moves to other strategies, such as direct mail, internet, point of sale, package branding and discounting. When regulation successfully eliminates all channels, the tobacco market will freeze up and dwindle over time. But we know that until every single channel for marketing is closed off, tobacco companies will try to spend their way around the problem because there is money to be made doing so. Thus, tobacco control must work relentlessly toward closing off every avenue available to tobacco companies to promote their destructive products. Such innovative anti-marketing efforts include requiring plain, standardized packaging of their products, and eventually plain, standardized products.

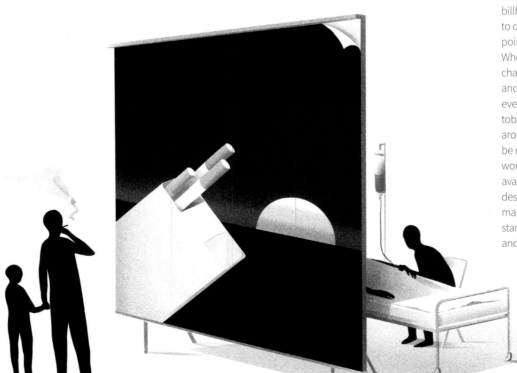

Advertising Bans
Total Number of Bans on Direct and Indirect Tobacco Advertising, 2016

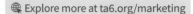 Explore more at ta6.org/marketing

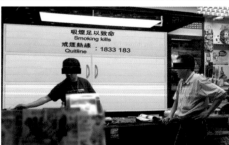

Legend:
- 13-16
- 9-12
- 5-9
- 0-5
- No Data
- Warning labels >50% of pack size
- Plain, standardized packaging and large graphic warning labels

BAD PRACTICE

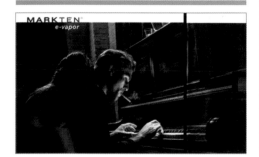

Surreptitious Promotion of Smoking Through E-Cigarette Adverts

Allowing for e-cigarettes ads that surreptitiously promote smoking in channels that are closed off to tobacco products. Philip Morris manufactures MarkTen e-cigarettes, which look nearly identical to cigarettes here as "smoke" floats off the end of the e-cigarette. Companies can claim they are only advertising e-cigarettes where cigarette ads have been banned, even though the products are indistinguishable to the viewer.

GOOD PRACTICE

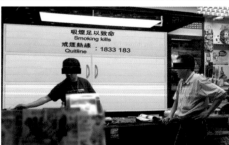

FCTC Compliance with Marketing Bans Across the Globe

This mockup of a bilingual point-of-sale advertising ban envisions what this policy would look like if adopted in Hong Kong. As of 2016, 15% of the world's population, living in 37 countries, were covered by the WHO FCTC's best-practice policy of banning tobacco advertising, promotion and sponsorship. Of the world population, 47% (in 78 countries) were covered by a tobacco health warning label that met best practices.

CUTTING EDGE PRACTICE

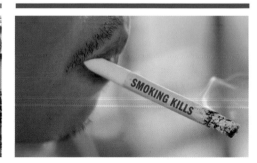

Plain, Standardized Packaging and Products

When tobacco companies responded to Australia's plain packaging law by adding distinctive markings to cigarettes, they were reprimanded as being "not strictly compliant" with current legislation. As a potentially important improvement on plain packaging legislation, Canada has considered standardizing the entire cigarette, going to a plain product, requiring wrapping the cigarette in an unpleasant color of paper.

CHAPTER 4

PREVALENCE

Percentage of Adult Males Who Smoke Daily
Age ≥10, 2015 or latest data available

🌐 Explore more at ta6.org/prevalence

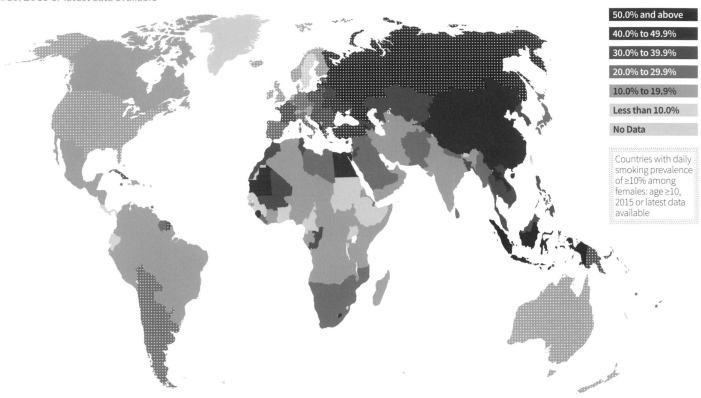

50.0% and above
40.0% to 49.9%
30.0% to 39.9%
20.0% to 29.9%
10.0% to 19.9%
Less than 10.0%
No Data

Countries with daily smoking prevalence of ≥10% among females: age ≥10, 2015 or latest data available

Globally, 942 million men and 175 million women ages 15 or older are current smokers. Nearly three quarters of male daily smokers live in countries with a medium or high human development index (HDI), whereas half of female daily smokers live in very high-HDI countries 📊.

Male smoking prevalence in most medium- to very high-HDI countries substantially increased in the past century, though this generally happened earlier in very high-HDI countries (the first half vs. second half of the 20th century). Almost all very high-HDI countries saw a significant decrease in male smoking after the 1950s. Many medium- or high-HDI countries have also seen a decline in prevalence, but mostly a relatively moderate one from the beginning of this century. Smoking prevalence has been historically modest in most low-HDI countries, though this still translates into tens of millions of smokers.

Female smoking prevalence in very high-HDI countries peaked a few decades later than the peak in male smoking, but it has remained relatively low or had a moderate increase thus far in other countries.

However, the earlier decreasing trend in smoking prevalence in most very high-HDI countries has stalled in recent years, and smoking prevalence has continued to rise or remained at high levels in many medium- or high-HDI countries. Further, some low-HDI countries (e.g., in sub-Saharan Africa) have seen a recent increase in prevalence 📊. This trend is likely to occur in many other low-HDI countries in the future because of income growth and increasing cigarette affordability, as well as the tobacco industry's strategy of aggressive marketing in those countries, unless governments implement stronger tobacco control policies, including raising taxes to increase prices of tobacco products.

Another major concern is a recent increase in smoking prevalence among youth, particularly among females, in several low- to high-HDI countries, in some of which smoking among adolescent girls is now more common than among adult women or even adolescent boys.

Nearly two thirds of countries, including 98% of low-HDI countries and 93% of countries in sub-Saharan Africa, have not implemented tobacco use monitoring at best-practice level 📊. Effective monitoring at the national level must be a priority for governments, as this is essential for estimating the tobacco-related burden and evaluating the success of tobacco control policies.

Although tobacco use remains a major health issue worldwide, the declines in prevalence in countries with active tobacco control efforts demonstrate that we can reduce smoking with effective strategies.

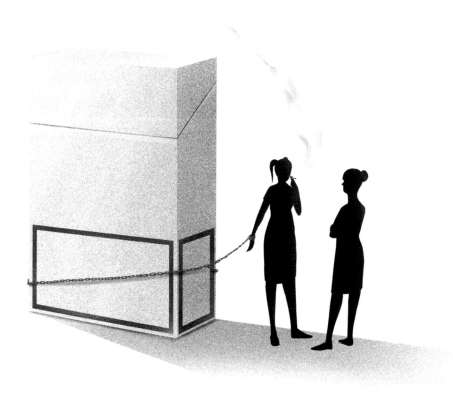

⊞ Global Distribution of Smokers

Three quarters of male daily smokers live in countries with medium or high-HDI, whereas half of female daily smokers live in very high-HDI countries

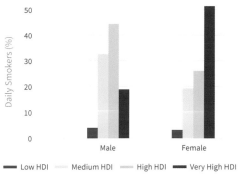

Low HDI ▬ Medium HDI ▬ High HDI ▬ Very High HDI

Male and female daily smokers globally, age ≥10 years, 2015, by country human development index

⊞ Recommended Level of Tobacco Monitoring

Many countries, particularly lower-HDI countries, lack an appropriate system for monitoring tobacco use

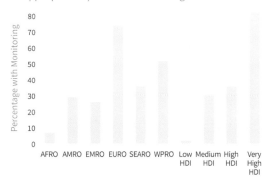

⊞ Smoking in Africa

Several sub-Saharan countries have seen a recent increase in smoking prevalence

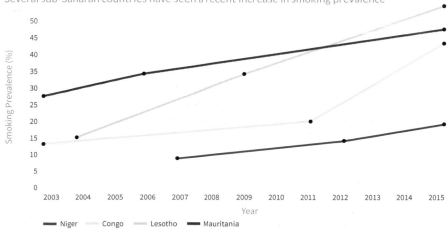

▬ Niger Congo Lesotho ▬ Mauritania

Trends in current tobacco smoking among males aged 15 years and over in select African countries

Changes in Consumption

Due to combination of population growth and increase in smoking rates, cigarette consumption in several WHO regions has substantially increased in recent decades

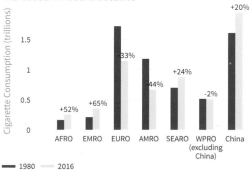

▬ 1980 ▬ 2016

Annual cigarette consumption and percentage of change 1980–2016, by WHO region

🌐 **Read the web-only chapter: ta6.org/consumption**

CHAPTER 6
HEALTH EFFECTS

Tobacco use is one of the most important preventable causes of premature death in the world. More than 6 million people per year die from tobacco use across the globe. There is no question that limiting tobacco use is one of the most effective ways to save lives and improve overall well-being.

Smoking tobacco causes exposure to a lethal mixture of more than 7000 toxic chemicals, including at least 70 known carcinogens that can damage nearly every organ system in the human body. Harms from tobacco begin before birth, as pregnant women who smoke give birth to infants at higher risk of congenital disorders, cancer, lung diseases, and sudden death. Newly identified risks from smoking include renal failure, intestinal ischemia, and hypertensive heart disease. The risk of death and disease from tobacco rises with the number of cigarettes smoked, but damage begins with use of a very small number of cigarettes. A regular life-long smoker loses at least 10–11 years of life to tobacco on average. In addition, exposure to second-hand or environmental tobacco smoke is associated with increased risk of cancer and heart disease, among other deleterious health effects.

Lung cancer is now the leading cause of cancer death in the world. It has long been the leading cause of cancer death among men, and in many countries is now also the leading cause of cancer death among women, outpacing breast cancer. Chronic obstructive pulmonary disease (COPD) is one of the leading causes of death in the world, and mortality from this condition is increasing in most countries; globally, 45% of all deaths from COPD are attributed to tobacco use. Similarly, death from heart disease and stroke, the two leading causes of death in the world, are heavily tied to tobacco use.

Combustible tobacco use is extremely hazardous to human health and is responsible for more than 90% of tobacco-attributable death and disease, despite efforts by the tobacco industry to market safer-sounding alternatives such as low-tar cigarettes and water pipes. Therefore, a top priority is to avoid combustible tobacco products, and the only way for an individual to completely eliminate tobacco-related harms is not to use them.

1. EYES
- Cataracts, blindness (macular degeneration)
- Stinging, excessive tearing and blinking

2. BRAIN AND PSYCHE
- Stroke (cerebrovascular accident)
- Addiction/withdrawal
- Altered brain chemistry
- Anxiety about tobacco's health effects

3. HAIR
- Odor and discoloration

4. NOSE
- Cancer of nasal cavities and paranasal sinuses
- Chronic rhinosinusitis
- Impaired sense of smell

5. TEETH
- Periodontal disease (gum disease, gingivitis, periodontitis)
- Loose teeth, tooth loss
- Root-surface caries, plaque
- Discoloration and staining

6. MOUTH AND THROAT
- Cancers of lips, mouth, throat, larynx and pharynx
- Sore throat
- Impaired sense of taste
- Bad breath

7. EARS
- Hearing loss
- Ear infection

8. LUNGS
- Lung, bronchus and tracheal cancer
- Chronic obstructive pulmonary disease (COPD) and emphysema
- Chronic bronchitis
- Respiratory infection (influenza, pneumonia, tuberculosis)
- Shortness of breath, asthma
- Chronic cough, excessive sputum production

9. HEART
- Coronary thrombosis (heart attack)
- Atherosclerosis (damage and occlusion of coronary vasculature)

10. CHEST & ABDOMEN
- Esophageal cancer
- Gastric, colon and pancreatic cancer
- Abdominal aortic aneurysm
- Peptic ulcer (esophagus, stomach, upper portion of small intestine)
- Possible increased risk of breast cancer

11. LIVER
- Liver cancer

12. MALE REPRODUCTION
- Infertility (sperm deformity, loss of motility, reduced number)
- Impotence
- Prostate cancer death

13. FEMALE REPRODUCTION
- Cervical and ovarian cancer
- Premature ovarian failure, early menopause
- Reduced fertility
- Painful menstruation

14. URINARY SYSTEM
- Bladder, kidney, and ureter cancer

15. HANDS
- Peripheral vascular disease, poor circulation (cold fingers)

16. SKIN
- Psoriasis
- Loss of skin tone, wrinkling, premature aging

17. SKELETAL SYSTEM
- Osteoporosis
- Hip fracture
- Susceptibility to back problems
- Bone marrow cancer
- Rheumatoid arthritis

18. WOUNDS AND SURGERY
- Impaired wound healing
- Poor post-surgical recovery
- Burns from cigarettes and from fires caused by cigarettes

19. LEGS AND FEET
- Peripheral vascular disease, cold feet, leg pain and gangrene
- Deep vein thrombosis

20. CIRCULATORY SYSTEM
- Buerger's disease (inflammation of arteries, veins and nerves in the legs)
- Acute myeloid leukemia

IMMUNE SYSTEM
- Impaired resistance to infection
- Possible increased risk of allergic diseases

OTHERS
- Diabetes
- Sudden death

Percent of DALYs Attributable to Tobacco Use

Tobacco use is responsible for a large proportion of disability-adjusted life years (DALYs) — the number of years lost due to ill-health, disability or early death

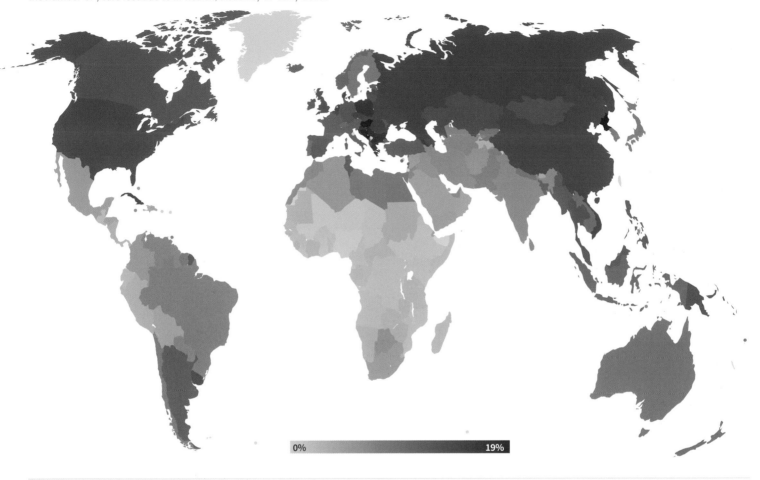

0%   19%

Deaths from Tobacco

Tobacco contributes to most of the leading causes of death in the world and half of all smokers will die from tobacco-related illness

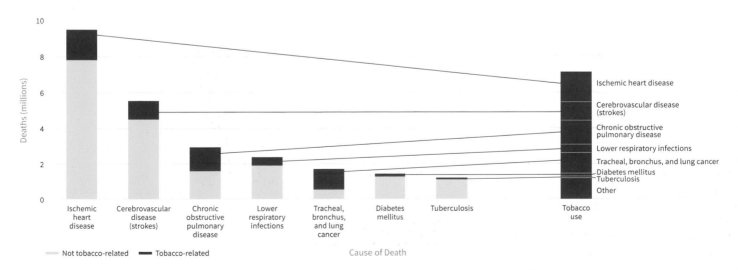

Not tobacco-related — Tobacco-related

Cause of Death

25

CHAPTER 7
COMORBIDITIES

Tuberculosis Mortality and Smoking

Independent of smoking, Africa already has among the largest TB challenges of any region, but models predict that smoking will greatly exacerbate TB mortality trends for the foreseeable future

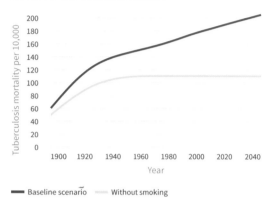

Baseline scenario — Without smoking

Smoking and HIV

As HIV-infected persons age, continued smoking robs them of more life than HIV-related factors

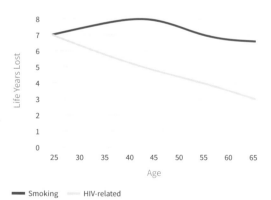

Smoking — HIV-related

I n the last several years, research has shown that the negative impacts that smoking has on health go far beyond lung cancer, chronic obstructive pulmonary disease (COPD), heart disease, stroke and other well-known consequences of tobacco use. We now know that tobacco helps fuel the global epidemic of tuberculosis, and it worsens problems such as mental illness, HIV infection and alcohol abuse.

Tuberculosis (TB) is the leading cause of death due to a single infectious agent in the world, and is the 6th-leading cause of death in the world overall, killing 1.8 million people in 2015. Cigarette smoking increases the risk of developing TB, and it makes treatment for TB less effective. Worldwide TB rates could decline as much as 20% if we eliminated smoking.

Persons with mental illness are more likely to smoke than people without such disorders, and it is much more difficult for them to quit. The more psychiatric diagnoses an individual patient has (among disorders such as schizophrenia, attention deficit disorder, bipolar illness, and others), the more likely it is that a person will smoke. For certain illnesses such as anxiety disorders, schizophrenia and bipolar illness, smoking seems to exacerbate symptoms, perhaps by making psychiatric medications less effective, and quitting smoking may improve symptoms as much as adding additional psychotropic drugs. In the US state of California, more than half of persons with mental disorders die from tobacco-related illness.

The harmful effects of smoking are magnified and accelerated in patients with HIV infection because when these patients use tobacco, they develop lung cancer and airway diseases such as COPD at higher rates and at younger ages than HIV-infected non-smokers. In settings where primary treatment for HIV infection is widely available and the disease can be well-managed, continuing tobacco use threatens progress in controlling AIDS, whereas in low-resource settings, it undermines already challenging treatment efforts even more.

Tuberculosis and Tobacco
Percentage of tuberculosis-related deaths due to tobacco

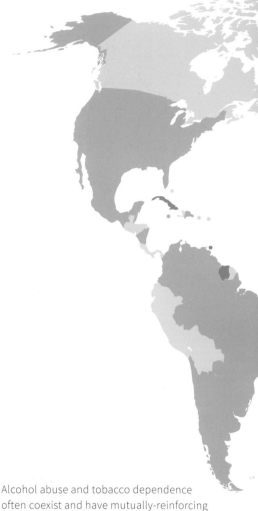

Alcohol abuse and tobacco dependence often coexist and have mutually-reinforcing harmful effects. A recent study in Russia demonstrated that although smoking was reported by "only" 14% of pregnant women, smoking prevalence was much higher (45%) among heavy drinkers and those at risk for an alcohol-exposed pregnancy. Thus, smoking and alcohol abuse co-occurred often and created a serious danger of dual prenatal exposure, with grave health consequences for offspring from those pregnancies.

Although links between tobacco and other serious medical conditions such as TB and HIV infection have been increasingly recognized, few TB or HIV clinics integrate smoking cessation programs into their routine services. This is an urgent need that must be addressed.

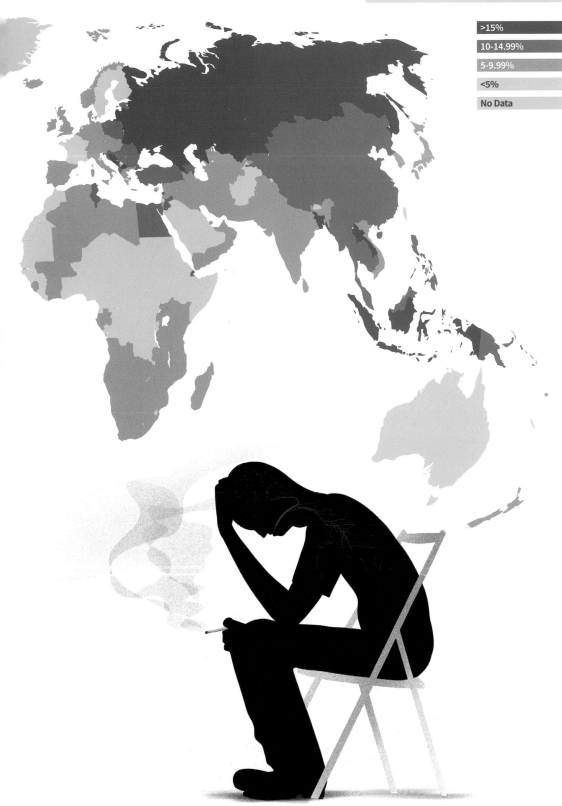

🌐 Explore more at ta6.org/comorbidities

Legend:
- >15%
- 10-14.99%
- 5-9.99%
- <5%
- No Data

Mental Illness and Adult Smoking in the United States

1 in 3

About 1 in 3 adults with mental illness smoke cigarettes (compared to 15% of adults with no mental illness)

3 in 10

Greater smoking intensity: about 3 in 10 cigarettes smoked by adults are smoked by adults with mental illness

1 in 5

Near 1 in 5 adults have some form of mental illness

CHAPTER 8

DEATHS

Deaths By Region

Number of tobacco-related deaths in the World Health Organization regions, all ages, 2016

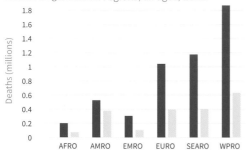

Deaths (millions)

- Male deaths
- Female deaths

Disparity in Tobacco Deaths

The burden of lung cancer deaths falls heaviest upon the least-educated

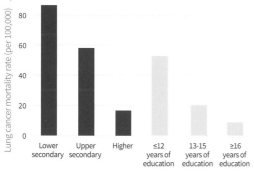

Lung cancer mortality rate (per 100,000)

Education Level Attained

- Poland (2011)
- United States, non-Hispanic whites (2010)

Percentage of Tobacco Deaths

Number of countries with percentage of deaths attributable to tobacco use, by WHO region, Males, all ages, 2016

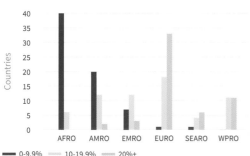

Countries

- 0-9.9%
- 10-19.9%
- 20%+

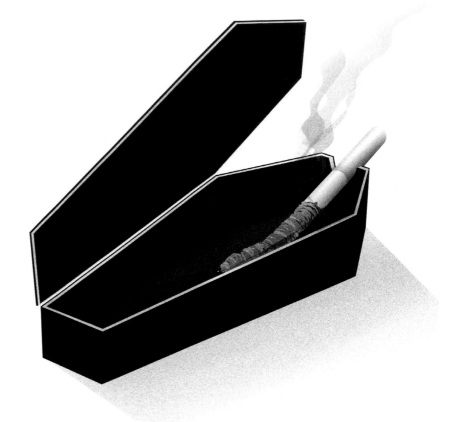

Tobacco use increases the risk of death from many diseases, including ischemic heart disease, cancer, stroke, and respiratory diseases. In 2016 alone, tobacco use caused over 7.1 million deaths worldwide (5.1 million in men, 2.0 million in women). Most of these deaths (6.3 million) were attributable to cigarette smoking, followed by secondhand smoke (884,000 deaths).

There is a several-decade lag between changes in smoking prevalence and changes in smoking-related death rates in the population. In general, countries with a very high human development index (HDI) have seen a decline in smoking prevalence at least since the 1960s, followed by a decrease in smoking-related death rates since the 1980s–90s. Nevertheless, the burden of smoking-related diseases, notably lung cancer, is still substantial in those countries. Smoking-related death rates are expected to increase for the decades to come

in many countries with a lower HDI, as they saw an increase in smoking prevalence more recently (the 1980s–90s or even later); in some, the prevalence is still increasing.

In about 55 countries, at least one-fifth of all deaths in males are attributable to smoking. These countries generally are high- or very high-HDI countries, mostly located in Europe (33 countries) or the Western Pacific region (11 countries), although there are two or more such countries in the other World Health Organization regions, except the African region. The lower tobacco-related burden in Sub-Saharan Africa reflects its historical lower smoking prevalence. However, with an increase in affordability of tobacco products and the tobacco industry's aggressive marketing in Africa, smoking prevalence has already started to rise, or is likely to substantially increase in the future. With its rapidly-growing populations and rising life expectancy, an increase in the number of

Deaths

Percentage of total male deaths attributable to tobacco

🌐 Explore more at ta6.org/deaths

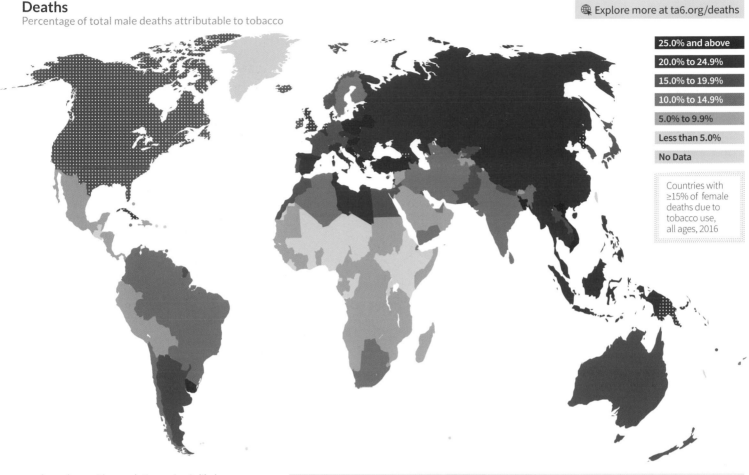

25.0% and above	
20.0% to 24.9%	
15.0% to 19.9%	
10.0% to 14.9%	
5.0% to 9.9%	
Less than 5.0%	
No Data	

Countries with ≥15% of female deaths due to tobacco use, all ages, 2016

smokers along with population aging is likely to make Africa suffer the most from future smoking-related burden.

Consistent with lower female smoking prevalence in many countries, the tobacco-related burden in women is lower than in men globally. However, with recent increases in smoking prevalence among female adolescents in some countries, this pattern may not continue.

In addition to very high-HDI countries, with current trends, most other countries are or will soon be facing substantial smoking-related burden, while many already have limited health resources. Even in very high-HDI countries, smoking prevalence and the related burden are now far higher among lower-income groups, which are more likely to have limited access to care 📊. This dynamic further underscores the need for effective tobacco control to improve health and reduce disparities at the population level in all countries.

📊 US Lung Cancer Deaths

Lung cancer is the leading cause of cancer deaths, accounting for at least one-fourth of all cancer deaths in both men and women in the United States

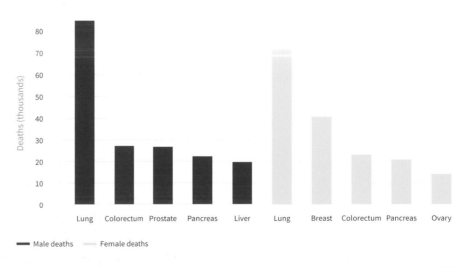

■ Male deaths ▬ Female deaths

Estimated number of cancer deaths for the leading five causes of cancer death by gender in the United States, 2017

SOCIETAL HARMS

Number of Smokers by HDI

The number of smokers is declining only in very-high HDI countries; in the rest of the world, the number of smokers is increasing

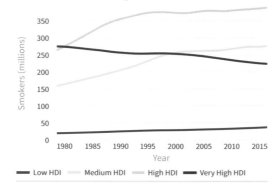

Smokers (millions) vs Year (1980–2015)

— Low HDI   — Medium HDI   — High HDI   — Very High HDI

Smoking Prevalence and Smoking-Related Mortality in Jamaica

The peak in smoking-related mortality lags behind the peak in smoking prevalence; smoking-related mortality can go up even if smoking prevalence declines

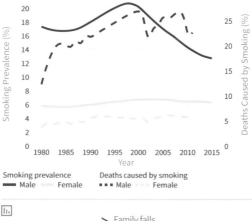

Smoking Prevalence (%) / Deaths Caused by Smoking (%) vs Year (1980–2015)

Smoking prevalence — Male — Female
Deaths caused by smoking ▪▪▪ Male ---- Female

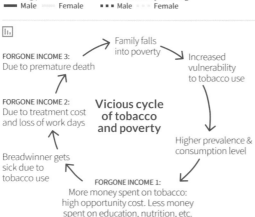

FORGONE INCOME 3:
Due to premature death

Family falls into poverty

Increased vulnerability to tobacco use

Vicious cycle of tobacco and poverty

Higher prevalence & consumption level

FORGONE INCOME 2:
Due to treatment cost and loss of work days

Breadwinner gets sick due to tobacco use

FORGONE INCOME 1:
More money spent on tobacco: high opportunity cost. Less money spent on education, nutrition, etc.

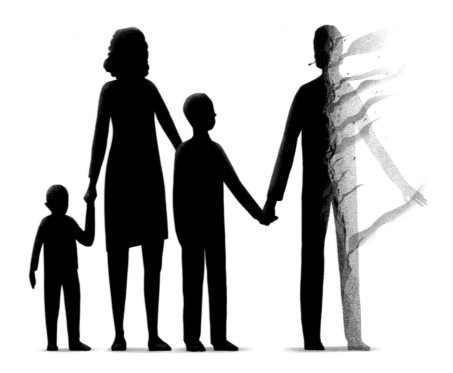

Tobacco-related harms reach far beyond the death and disease caused by tobacco consumption. Put simply, tobacco harms the world's sustainable development. The economic cost of smoking globally amounts to nearly 2 trillion dollars (in 2016 purchasing power parity) each year, equivalent to almost 2% of the world's total economic output. The majority of the total economic cost of smoking is the lost productivity of those sickened or killed by tobacco. Another 30% of these costs are the healthcare-related expenses of treating smoking-attributable diseases. Notably, this price tag does not include other substantial costs, such as the costs caused by second-hand smoke, non-combustible tobacco products, the environmental and health damages from tobacco farming, smoking-related fire hazards, cigarette butt littering, and, foremost, the immeasurable pain and suffering of tobacco victims and their families.

The cost of tobacco use is rising rapidly, following the increase in the number of tobacco users in low-, medium-, and high-HDI countries. Given the limited resources in most countries, these costs represent a lost opportunity to instead spend these resources on advancing the economy through education, healthcare, technology, and manufacturing. Because most health effects of smoking lag smoking initiation by more than a decade, the societal harm of smoking will still inevitably increase in countries where tobacco consumption has risen, and even in those where it has only recently started to fall.

Most tobacco users become addicted as youth without knowing the health consequences that tobacco use will eventually inflict upon them in the future, causing a level of economic hardship that they would undoubtedly not have chosen for their families or themselves. Regardless of a country's stage of economic development, the

Economic Cost of Smoking-Attributable Diseases

🌐 Explore more at ta6.org/societal-harms

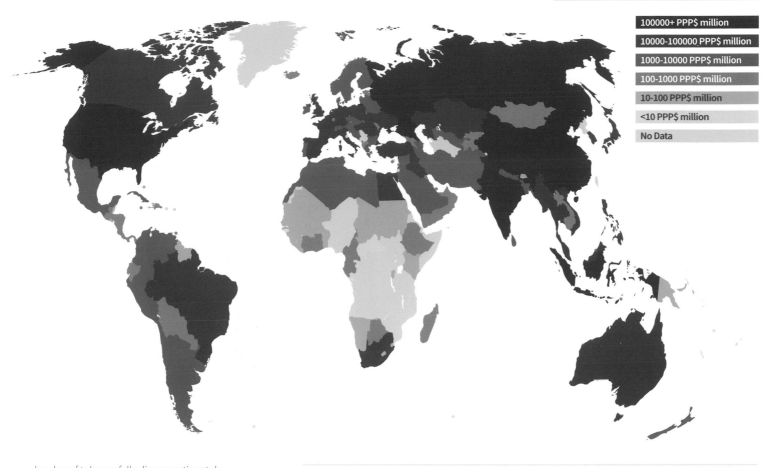

Legend:
- 100000+ PPP$ million
- 10000-100000 PPP$ million
- 1000-10000 PPP$ million
- 100-1000 PPP$ million
- 10-100 PPP$ million
- <10 PPP$ million
- No Data

burden of tobacco falls disproportionately on the poor, and is a source of both health and economic disparities 📊. The poor spend a larger share of their income on tobacco products, crowding out spending on necessities such as food, education, health and shelter. Additionally, tobacco-related illnesses contribute to catastrophic health expenditures that compete with basic needs in poor households. When a family breadwinner gets sick or dies prematurely due to tobacco use, the entire family is devastated and further impoverished. This cycle of tobacco use and poverty is vicious 📊 and will perpetuate through generations without intensified tobacco control efforts; thus, there is a particular need for efforts directed toward the poor.

The following chapters of the Atlas will focus on proven tobacco control strategies. The development and implementation of these strategies are fundamental investments in human capital that promotes human development.

📊 Disparities in Smoking Prevalence

In both men and women, differences in smoking prevalence can contribute to overall health and economic disparities

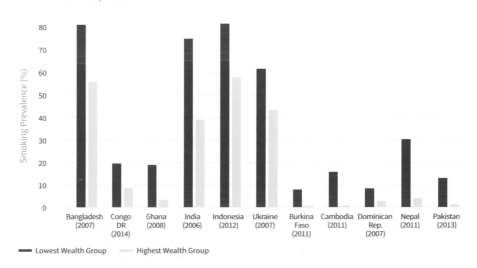

Smoking Prevalence (%)

Categories: Bangladesh (2007), Congo DR (2014), Ghana (2008), India (2006), Indonesia (2012), Ukraine (2007), Burkina Faso (2011), Cambodia (2011), Dominican Rep. (2007), Nepal (2011), Pakistan (2013)

— Lowest Wealth Group   — Highest Wealth Group

THE
SOLU

TION

CHAPTER 10
GLOBAL STRATEGY

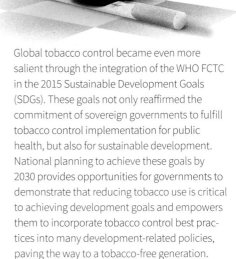

📊 Tobacco Control in Global Development

Tobacco control is not limited to the target of reducing the burden of tobacco-related diseases; it is an integral part of the global development agenda

UNITED NATIONS

SUSTAINABLE DEVELOPMENT GOAL

Ensure healthy lives and promote well being

UNITED NATIONS

NON-COMMUNICABLE DISEASE TARGET

By 2030, reduce premature mortality from non-communicable diseases by one third

WORLD HEALTH ORGANIZATION

SPECIFIC SMOKING PREVALENCE TARGET

Reduce tobacco use prevalence 30% by 2025. Implement WHO FCTC-compliant comprehensive tobacco control program.

Increased revenue from tobacco tax increases available financing for health and development

To address the tobacco menace more successfully, there have been important, over-arching global efforts to promote tobacco control. One of the central initiatives to situate country-level efforts in the global context has been the World Health Organization Framework Convention on Tobacco Control (WHO FCTC), which came into force in 2005 and provides a systematic framework of obligations and corresponding guidelines to reach tobacco control success. The ratification of this international treaty is voluntary and draws upon the political commitment of signatory countries to develop, implement and enforce the interventions. As of late 2017, the treaty had 181 Parties. For many, it provides effective political acceptability to implement politically-challenging measures.

The implementation of key tobacco control demand-reduction measures (e.g., tobacco taxation; smoke-free policies; packaging and labeling provisions; marketing bans; and cessation programs) at the highest levels of achievement accelerated among the WHO FCTC Parties between 2007 and 2014 📊. Effective implementation of these measures is significantly associated with lower smoking prevalence, which typically leads to considerable reductions in tobacco-related morbidity and mortality.

Global tobacco control also fits snugly into broader public health efforts, for example by constituting a major element of the United Nations' efforts to address noncommunicable diseases (NCDs) around the world 📊. The 2012 Political Declaration of the High-Level Meeting of the United Nations General Assembly (UNGA) recognized the enormous health and economic burden of NCDs on households and nations, and agreed to reduce deaths from four prominent NCDs (i.e. cancer, diabetes, lung disease and cardiovascular disease) 📍. The WHO created voluntary targets for prevention of premature deaths from these NCDs, which includes a 30% relative reduction in adult smoking prevalence 📊.

Global tobacco control became even more salient through the integration of the WHO FCTC in the 2015 Sustainable Development Goals (SDGs). These goals not only reaffirmed the commitment of sovereign governments to fulfill tobacco control implementation for public health, but also for sustainable development. National planning to achieve these goals by 2030 provides opportunities for governments to demonstrate that reducing tobacco use is critical to achieving development goals and empowers them to incorporate tobacco control best practices into many development-related policies, paving the way to a tobacco-free generation.

Momentum is also building globally— including from organizations such as the World Bank— to use tobacco tax revenue for financing poverty alleviation and other development programs critical to many resource-poor countries 📊. With the opportunity to generate significant revenue while reducing tobacco consumption and tobacco-induced health and environmental costs, tobacco taxation can stand out as a win-win policy for development (see text below.)

The Success Story of the Sin Tax Reform in the Philippines

Enacted in December 2012, the reform was anchored to financing the expansion of Universal Health Care (UHC), in addition to alternative livelihood programs for tobacco farmers and health promotion. More than 85% of the incremental revenue from excise on tobacco and alcohol products was dedicated to these programs. Smoking prevalence declined sharply and the increased revenue helped to nearly triple the number of poor people with free health insurance coverage in three years.

♀ The Toll of NCDs on Humanity
Share of total deaths due to NCDs (%), 2016

⊕ Explore more at ta6.org/global-strategy

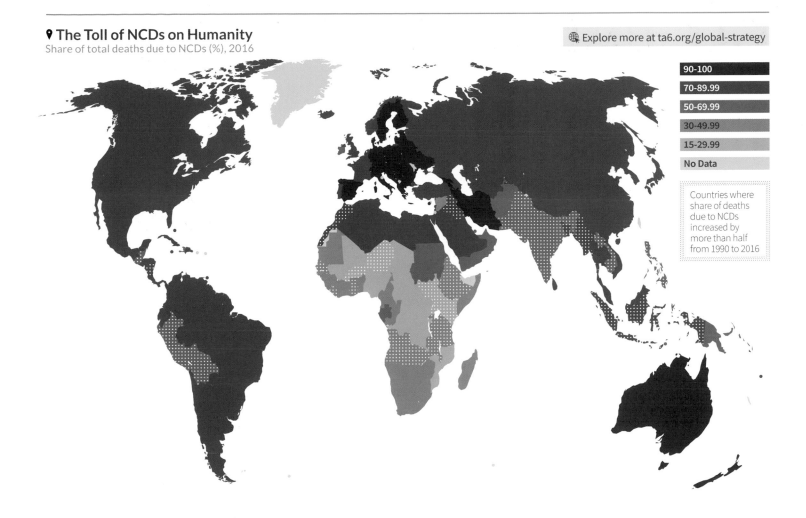

■	90-100
■	70-89.99
■	50-69.99
■	30-49.99
■	15-29.99
■	No Data

Countries where share of deaths due to NCDs increased by more than half from 1990 to 2016

▥ Progress in Tobacco Demand-Reduction Measures

The implementation of key tobacco control demand-reduction measures at the highest level of achievement accelerated among the WHO FCTC Parties between 2007 and 2014

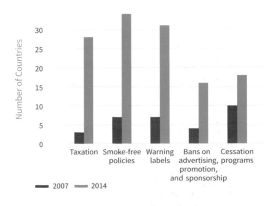

Number of Countries

Taxation | Smoke-free policies | Warning labels | Bans on advertising, promotion, and sponsorship | Cessation programs

— 2007 — 2014

▥ Tobacco Taxes to Aid Tobacco Control as well as Development

The annual increase in global excise revenue by $190 billion PPP, from raising cigarette excise tax in each country by $1 PPP per 20-cigarette pack, could lift a quarter of the world's 767 million poor above the poverty line

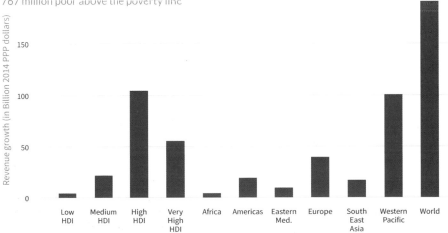

Revenue growth (in Billion 2014 PPP dollars)

Low HDI | Medium HDI | High HDI | Very High HDI | Africa | Americas | Eastern Med. | Europe | South East Asia | Western Pacific | World

CHAPTER 11
QUITTING

📊 Smokers Want to Quit

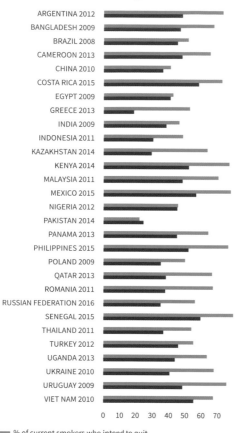

ARGENTINA 2012
BANGLADESH 2009
BRAZIL 2008
CAMEROON 2013
CHINA 2010
COSTA RICA 2015
EGYPT 2009
GREECE 2013
INDIA 2009
INDONESIA 2011
KAZAKHSTAN 2014
KENYA 2014
MALAYSIA 2011
MEXICO 2015
NIGERIA 2012
PAKISTAN 2014
PANAMA 2013
PHILIPPINES 2015
POLAND 2009
QATAR 2013
ROMANIA 2011
RUSSIAN FEDERATION 2016
SENEGAL 2015
THAILAND 2011
TURKEY 2012
UGANDA 2013
UKRAINE 2010
URUGUAY 2009
VIET NAM 2010

0 10 20 30 40 50 60 70

— % of current smokers who intend to quit
— % of current smokers who attempted to quit in past 12 months

📊 Declines In Risk After Quitting

Former smokers who stop smoking by about 40 years old reduce their risk of dying from lung cancer by 90%

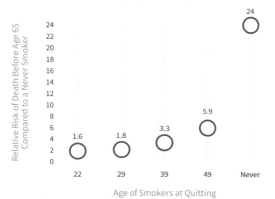

Relative Risk of Death Before Age 65 Compared to a Never Smoker

24
22
20
18
16
14
12
10
8
6
4
2
0

24

5.9

3.3

1.6   1.8

22   29   39   49   Never

Age of Smokers at Quitting

Quitting tobacco use benefits health at any age. For smokers, smoking cessation is one of the best ways to add years to their lives. The benefits of quitting occur almost instantly 📊 and most smokers want to quit smoking 📊. But quitting is difficult for most smokers, and the majority make multiple quit attempts during their lifetime, during which time they are losing life-years. Moreover, tobacco cessation is a cost-effective healthcare intervention. Accordingly, governments and healthcare providers should make available more and accessible resources to help tobacco users stop, as enshrined in the WHO FCTC Article 14. However, most governments are failing would-be quitters 📍.

It is important to reach young smokers with cessation messages and aids. The younger someone is when they stop smoking, the greater the benefit in terms of years of life saved. Smoking causes a decade of life lost, but quitting before the age of 40 can essentially return 9 of those years on average, because cessation by that age reduces a former smoker's chance of death from tobacco-related illness by 90% 📊. At the same time, getting adult smokers to stop helps population health almost immediately.

The healthcare system and healthcare workers should be on the frontline of tobacco cessation. They can reach many tobacco users directly, interact regularly with them particularly at key life moments (e.g., disease diagnosis, pregnancy, etc.), and are typically a trusted information source. Using existing health infrastructure, the strategy is also economical. Cessation should be integrated into health professionals' work by training them to 1) ask individuals if they smoke and record this, 2) advise smokers to stop, and 3) actively offer help for quitting. Currently, less than half of countries even help health workers to quit or integrate tobacco cessation into basic medical advisement, and less than a third mandate recording tobacco use in patient notes.

Currently, there are too few examples of successful population-level cessation strategies. Governments must invest in promoting cessation, by developing evidence-based national strategies and guidelines, and allocating sufficient implementation resources. Governments can introduce and maintain national quitlines, promote and support counseling for quitters (including mobile phone text messaging services), make cessation medicines more accessible and affordable, and establish mass communication programs to promote quitting. In 2017, only a quarter of WHO FCTC parties had a clearly-identified budget for cessation, and less than a quarter had a free, national quitline. Moreover, with only a few exceptions 📍, lower-HDI countries are struggling most to develop cessation strategies. Raising tobacco taxes pairs well with these efforts: higher taxes promote quitting, and a fraction of new tax revenue could support quitting programs.

⚲ WHO Cessation Index

⊕ Explore more at ta6.org/quitting

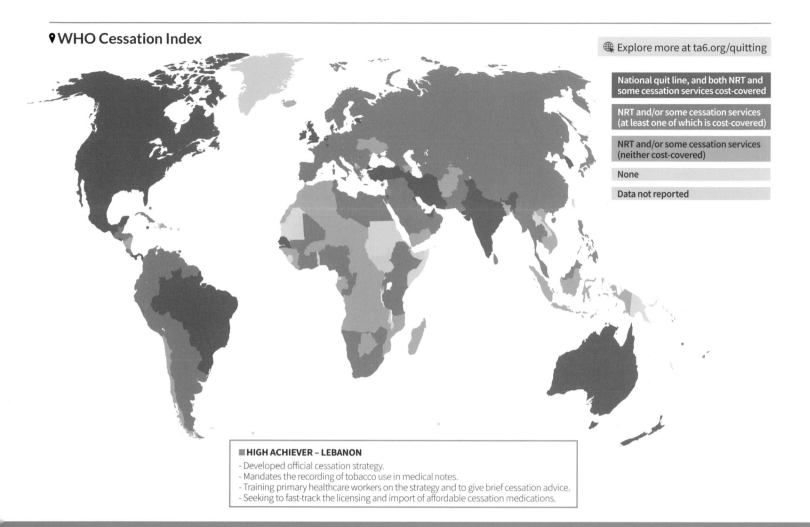

National quit line, and both NRT and some cessation services cost-covered

NRT and/or some cessation services (at least one of which is cost-covered)

NRT and/or some cessation services (neither cost-covered)

None

Data not reported

■ **HIGH ACHIEVER – LEBANON**
- Developed official cessation strategy.
- Mandates the recording of tobacco use in medical notes.
- Training primary healthcare workers on the strategy and to give brief cessation advice.
- Seeking to fast-track the licensing and import of affordable cessation medications.

📊 Effects of Quitting Over Time

WITHIN **20** MINUTES	WITHIN **12** HOURS	WITHIN **2-12** WEEKS	WITHIN **1-9** MONTHS	WITHIN **1** YEAR	WITHIN **5** YEARS	WITHIN **10** YEARS	WITHIN **15** YEARS
Your heart rate and blood pressure drop.	Your carbon monoxide level in the blood drops to normal.	Your circulation improves and your lung function increases.	Your coughing and shortness of breath decrease.	Your risk of coronary heart disease is about half that of a smoker's.	Your risk of stroke is reduced to that of a nonsmoker's.	Your risk of lung cancer falls to about half that of a smoker's, and your risk of cancer of the mouth, throat, esophagus, bladder, cervix, or pancreas decreases.	Your risk of coronary heart disease is that of a nonsmoker's.

TAXES

📊 Meeting the WHO 30% Prevalence Reduction Target Globally

Tobacco tax increases that result in higher tobacco product prices are among the most effective tobacco control measures available

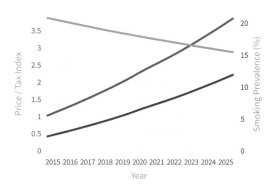

— Price **—** Tax **—** Prevalence

Making cigarettes four times more costly in all countries globally by 2025 would reduce the world's tobacco use prevalence from the current 21% to 15% in 2025. Such a drop in prevalence would be sufficient to reach the World Health Organization target of reducing tobacco use prevalence 30% by 2025. This scenario is attainable, but would require a 7-fold excise tax increase.

Differential Tax Treatment Can Lead to Product Substitution

Cigarette and roll-your-own tobacco sales in Cyprus

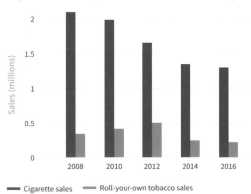

— Cigarette sales **—** Roll-your-own tobacco sales

When the 2008-2012 cigarette excise tax increases made cigarettes more expensive in Cyprus, some tobacco users quit, while others switched to relatively cheaper roll-your-own tobacco. Only after a substantial tax increase on roll-your-own tobacco had reduced the price difference between the two products in 2013, did the sales of both cigarettes and roll-your-own tobacco decline.

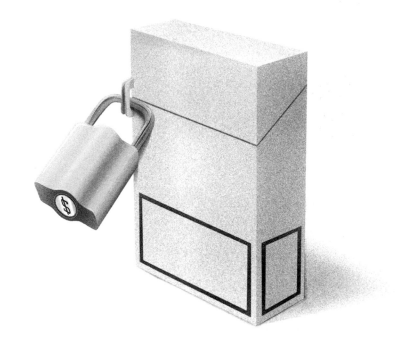

When thinking about stopping an epidemic, tax is usually not the first thing that comes to mind. Yet perhaps the most impactful way to reduce tobacco use is to tax tobacco products. Some countries are already successfully using tax to reduce smoking rates, reaping significant and immediate health and revenue benefits. While there is no maximum tax level, some set ambitious goals, such as New Zealand's goal to increase the cost of a cigarette pack to 30 New Zealand dollars (ca. 20 USD) through excise taxation. Unfortunately, most of the world, predominantly its poorer parts, still lags in implementing high tobacco taxes 📊 📍.

The mechanisms behind tobacco taxation are simple. A sufficiently large tax increase will raise tobacco product prices. By observing smokers' behavior, researchers have determined that on average a 10% increase in cigarette prices makes the consumption of cigarettes fall by between 2% and 8%. Higher tobacco prices are especially effective in reducing tobacco use in more vulnerable populations, such as youth and lower-income people, because those groups are particularly sensitive to price increases 🌐. Frequent, significant tax increases are especially needed in countries where consumer purchasing power is growing. When incomes rise faster than cigarette prices, smoking becomes more affordable, encouraging consumption 🌐. Excise tax increases are a proven and effective way to make cigarettes and other tobacco products less affordable.

Globally, we have yet to realize significant opportunities for improving health from tobacco taxation. For example, using only tobacco taxes, countries could realistically achieve the World Health Organization target of a 30% relative reduction in smoking prevalence by 2025 📊. Unfortunately, many governments are still reluctant to increase taxes, because they often rely on tobacco industry reports that typically suggest that any additional tax increase will cause declines in tax revenue or a massive increase in cigarette smuggling. Independent studies have shown that these claims are usually greatly exaggerated; new tax increases bring in additional revenue for the governments, whereas illicit trade in tobacco products can be controlled while keeping prices high 📊. When in force, the Protocol to Eliminate Illicit Trade in Tobacco Products will provide powerful tools to combat cigarette smuggling globally.

🌐 **Read more at ta6.org/illicit-trade**

Cigarette Prices

Price of 20-cigarette pack of the most-sold brand in US dollars; adjusted for purchasing power of national currencies

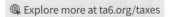 Explore more at ta6.org/taxes

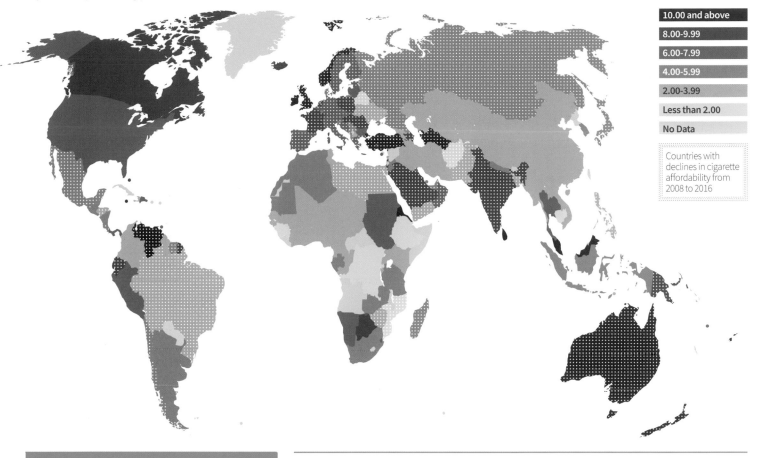

■	10.00 and above
■	8.00-9.99
■	6.00-7.99
■	4.00-5.99
■	2.00-3.99
■	Less than 2.00
■	No Data

Countries with declines in cigarette affordability from 2008 to 2016

Share of the World's Population Covered by Different Cigarette Tax Levels, 2016

While there is no maximum tax level:

1 in 100
people live in countries with no cigarette excise tax.

4 in 10
people are covered only by minimal cigarette taxes – i.e., total tax below 50% of the retail cigarette price.

Only

1 in 10
people are covered by tax at or above the WHO minimum-recommended 75% of the retail cigarette price.

Tax increases Do Not Lead to Increased Cigarette Smuggling

Cigarette prices vs. illicit market in the UK

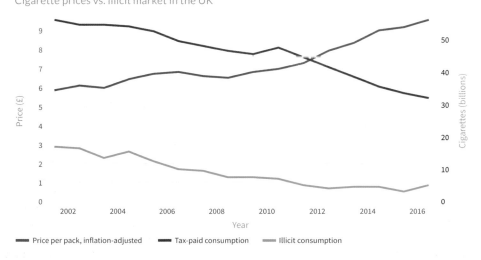

— Price per pack, inflation-adjusted   — Tax-paid consumption   — Illicit consumption

Due to periodic cigarette tax increases, the inflation-adjusted price of cigarettes in the UK increased by 63% from 2001 to 2016, making UK cigarette prices among the highest in the world. At the same time, the illicit market dropped by over 70%, along with dropping tax-paid consumption.

CHAPTER 13

SMOKE-FREE

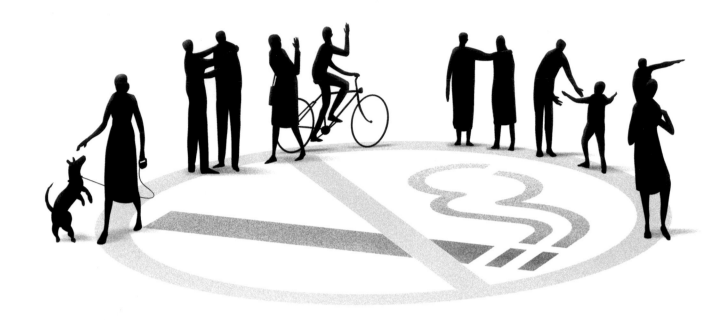

📊 Progress in Smoke-free Legislation 2007-2016

Current global population: 7.6 billion

[Chart with left axis "Population protected (billions)" ranging 0 to 8.0, right axis "Countries" ranging 0 to 150, showing years 2007, 2008, 2010, 2012, 2014, 2016]

— Countries — Population

📊 What is thirdhand smoke?

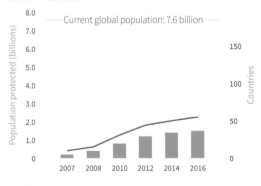

It refers to residues of tobacco and tobacco byproducts that solidify and form in carpets, drapes, and other surfaces in rooms where smoking occurred. These residues contain many of the harmful substances found in tobacco smoke itself.

Creating smoke-free environments is a vital tobacco control intervention and serves important purposes. First and foremost, these laws protect non-smokers from the harmful effects of second-hand and even thirdhand smoke 📊. Secondhand smoke has been associated with most of the same harmful health effects as direct smoking. Conversely, one study of bartenders documented prompt improvements in lung function after indoor smoking bans were enacted. Second, limiting smoking in public places helps to create the sense that smoking is socially unacceptable behavior, and reinforces the idea of non-smoking as a societal norm. Smokers who cannot smoke in public are also more likely to try to quit.

At present, despite some progress 📊, most of the world's population is currently left unprotected by strong smoke-free laws and regulations. National-level bans exist in some countries, such as Turkey, which passed a ban in 2008 prohibiting tobacco use in all indoor spaces including bars, cafés and restaurants, sports stadia, and the gardens of mosques and hospitals. Sometimes, laws that are in place have been enacted locally. In New York City,

for example, smoking is not allowed in bars, restaurants, clubs, public parks, city beaches, or even apartments in public housing projects. Although approximately 1.5 billion people around the world are now protected to some extent by smoking bans in public places, more than 80% of the world's population is still vulnerable to secondhand smoke.

In many countries and cities, smoking in many public places (e.g., airports) is only allowed in specially designated smoking rooms. Such partial bans are often ineffective. Ventilation for such smoking rooms does not remove all the smoke, so leakage occurs around doors and windows. Additionally, smoking is still preserved as a social norm, removing a major motivating factor for smokers to quit 📊.

Governments must be comprehensive and forceful in their smoke-free policies. For example, some jurisdictions have begun to include water pipes in their ban, or have at least implemented partial bans (e.g., the United Arab Emirates). E-cigarette public bans (including New York City) — not without controversy — have also become more common around the globe.

Smoke-free Environments

Countries with all public places completely smoke-free (or at least 90% of the population covered by complete subnational smoke-free legislation)

🌐 Explore more at ta6.org/smoke-free

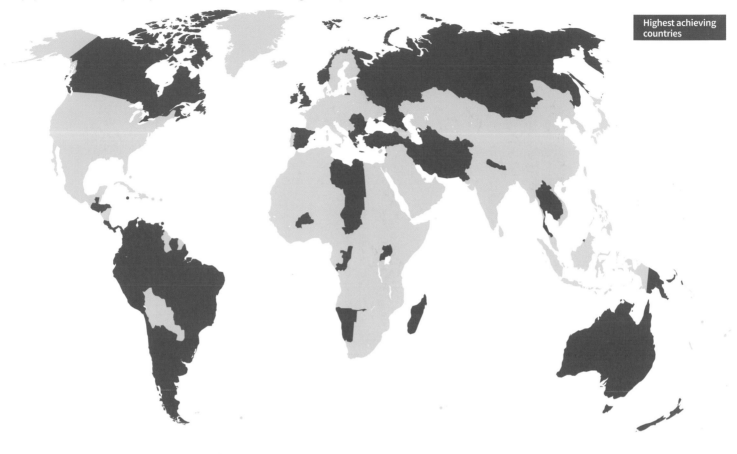

Highest achieving countries

📊 BAD PRACTICE

Designated smoking areas leak smoke and make public smoking acceptable

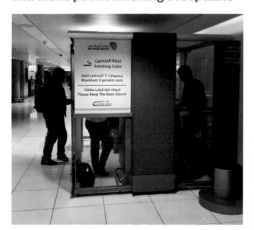

GOOD PRACTICE

Smoking outlawed in tram stations in Turkey

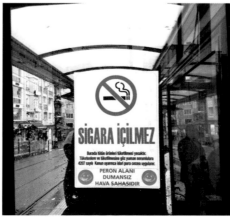

BEST PRACTICES

- Prohibit smoking in all indoor public places, indoor workplaces, and public transport, without exception (including the elimination of designated smoking areas).

- Policies should be comprehensive to include products such as water pipes and cigars that sometimes receive special treatment.

- Monitor compliance and strengthen enforcement. Consider including administrative sanctions for establishments not in compliance (such as revocation of licenses).

- Expand the list of outdoor (e.g., stadia) and semi-outdoor places (e.g., covered patios) where smoking is prohibited.

41

CHAPTER 14
MEDIA CAMPAIGNS

As individuals' knowledge and belief in the toxic health effects of tobacco use grow, the likelihood of using tobacco decreases and their support for protective policies increases. Mass media give us the opportunity to efficiently persuade large populations about the urgent need for action. Using media to inspire individuals to quit tobacco or persuade them not to start using it, and societies to take up policies for a tobacco-free future is a critical part of the tobacco control toolbox.

Media campaigns are embedded both in both WHO FCTC Article 12 and the WHO MPOWER package – "W" for Warning. Successful campaigns change individual behavior, shift broader social norms, and build popular support for tobacco control policies. Moreover, research in countries across the Human Development Index (HDI) demonstrates that campaigns can be cost-effective — just a few cents per quit attempt in some countries 📊.

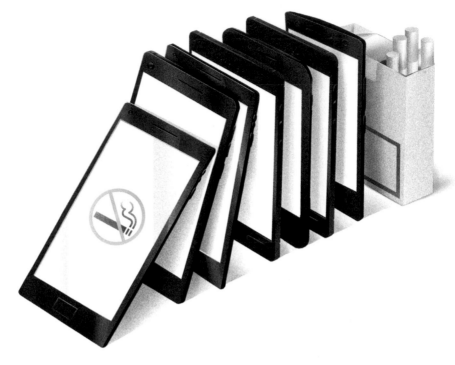

Two essential components of successful campaigns are effective messaging and delivery. Research consistently demonstrates the effectiveness of campaigns that challenge audiences to deal with the specific negative impacts of smoking — e.g., cancer, blindness and lung disease. Some examples are victims' real-world testimonials or graphic depictions of damage.

Best-practice campaigns use behavioral research to test messages with intended audiences— e.g., male smokers— to ensure they are effective and culturally relevant. In lower-HDI countries, costly research can be avoided by adapting campaigns from other areas that have a strong evidence of success and target similar populations— e.g., compelling graphic images have been found to have wide application across many cultures. Supportive campaign messages such as highlighting stories of happy ex-smokers may also reinforce smokers' belief they can successfully quit. A poorly-messaged campaign can have little or no impact. Finally, it is critical to rigorously evaluate a campaign's impact.

Underinvestment in media delivery and planning is a frequent failing of tobacco control programs.

Successful use of mass media requires sustained campaigns with broad population reach. This includes keeping campaigns "on the air" most months of the year. The most successful campaigns use a mix of media channels— usually television and radio due to their high reach and proven impact —with social and digital media as an emerging tool in many key populations 📊. Sustained media delivery with high reach, such as extended national television campaigns, can be expensive. Many countries have implemented innovative policies to ensure that their tobacco control media campaigns receive placements. These range from health promotion foundations that utilize tobacco taxes to fund campaigns to legislation that mandates television and radio channels dedicate a portion of prime-time programming to public health messages 📊.

Recent evidence shows that campaigns can use social media to mobilize large populations to advocate for tobacco control policies. In Vietnam, small-dollar social media ads on Facebook were used to generate significant public discourse online and offline around pending legislation, which ultimately passed.

📊 Impressive return on investment for media campaigns in India

QUIT ATTEMPT	**USD 0.06**
PERMANENT QUIT	**USD 2.60**
DEATH AVERTED	**USD 9.20**

Mass Media and Quitting
Mass media campaigns have prompted increases in quit line calls and turned the tide of public support for novel policies

The national "Sponge" mass media campaign in Senegal prompted a near 600% increase in calls to the quit line, compared to the pre-campaign period.

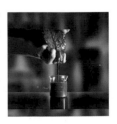

Mass Media Best Practice Countries

High- and low-HDI countries have mounted gold-standard media campaigns, but globally media campaigns remain underutilized

🌐 Explore more at ta6.org/media-campaigns

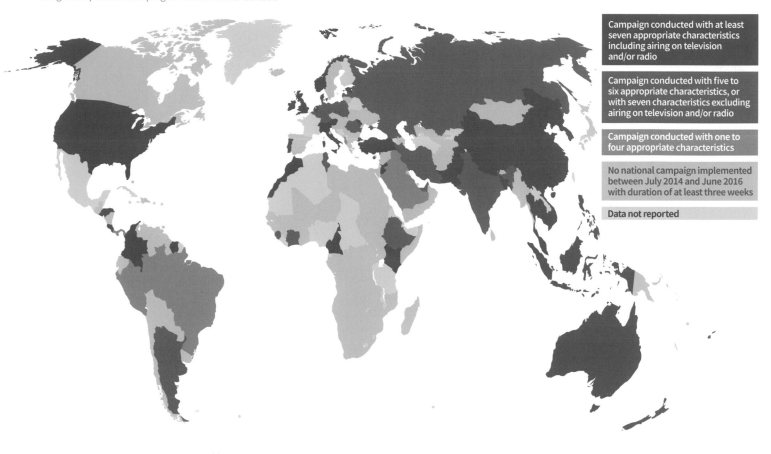

- Campaign conducted with at least seven appropriate characteristics including airing on television and/or radio
- Campaign conducted with five to six appropriate characteristics, or with seven characteristics excluding airing on television and/or radio
- Campaign conducted with one to four appropriate characteristics
- No national campaign implemented between July 2014 and June 2016 with duration of at least three weeks
- Data not reported

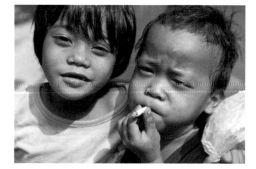

BAD PRACTICE

Anti-tobacco education initiatives that are based within schools have been found to be largely ineffectual. The most impactful campaigns have been shown to be those using mass media to target large segments of the population, with hard-hitting messages on the harms of tobacco for most months of the year.

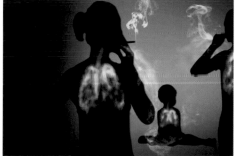

📊 GOOD PRACTICE

Australia's long-running efforts using mass media have helped drive down tobacco use to record lows among adults and youth. The country's sustained effort uses television, radio and digital platforms to achieve greater population reach and has produced graphic advertising that has been adapted around the world.

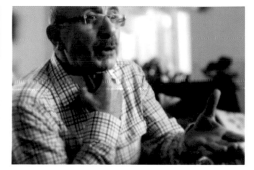

📊 CUTTING EDGE PRACTICE

Turkey's comprehensive tobacco control legislation requires TV and radio stations to air 90 minutes of Ministry of Health ads each month, including 30 minutes in peak hours. Using this innovative strategy, Turkey has mounted numerous anti-tobacco campaigns each year, reaching most citizens and driving millions to quit smoking.

CHAPTER 15

PARTNERSHIPS

The complexities of tobacco control interventions necessitate collaboration among a multitude of actors. Challenged by systematic tobacco industry interference, a wide range of local, regional and international civil society partners, international health and development governmental organizations, local and national government ministries, and private businesses have partnered together to confront and counter the tobacco industry. The results to date have been a mix of many different types of partnerships and a growing body of evidence of what works and what does not.

For 16 years, Vital Strategies (VS) and the American Cancer Society (ACS) have worked together to produce this important resource, *The Tobacco Atlas*, for the public health community. In hindsight, the fruits of this enduring partnership can be largely attributed to an alignment of interests, skills and needs between the two organizations. More specifically, they both:

• Are passionate about tobacco control and see the value in the resource they are producing;
• Bring different yet complementary skills and expertise to the partnership;
• Have strong subject matter expertise and similar enough views on issues that allow them to avoid major differences of opinion or find acceptable and appropriate compromises;

• Bring resources to the partnership making neither wholly dependent on the other;
• Like, trust, and appreciate each other; and
• Can make key decisions together and follow timelines effectively.

A recent outcome from this successful partnership is that the two organizations have banded together again to support the global cancer community in their efforts to raise the profile of tobacco taxation as a cancer prevention strategy through the Prevent20 Coalition ♀.

Among other things, ACS and VS plan to monitor progress and outcomes to share successes and lessons learned from the partnership and encourage other risk factor and disease-focused groups to emulate achievements for further impact.

Each day there are new opportunities to innovate as a tobacco control community that require less-traditional partnerships to address important evolving issues. Establishing stronger linkages among the tobacco control, global health and development communities has been recognized as an important priority. Regulating new tobacco products also presents a complex set of challenges that will require sustained collaborative and cooperative efforts.

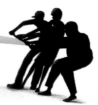

Brazil – Partnering to Counter Tobacco Industry Tactics

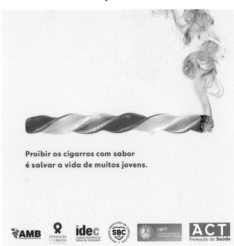

Proibir os cigarros com sabor é salvar a vida de muitos jovens.

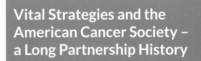

In Brazil, the tobacco industry has systematically interfered with tobacco control legislation, most recently halting the progress of Brazil's ban on tobacco additives. To counter this interference, prominent health NGOs allied under the auspices of the national tobacco control coalition worked with government agencies and unlikely partners, like tobacco farmer organizations, to engage in sustained and strategic advocacy efforts. They also received instrumental international support from the Bloomberg Initiative to Reduce Tobacco Use partners.

Vital Strategies and the American Cancer Society – a Long Partnership History

COMMON OBJECTIVE: TOBACCO CONTROL POLICY ADVOCACY

 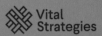

Research, global programs   Strategic communications & media relations

The American Cancer Society, via its Research and Global Cancer Control departments, has been partnering with Vital Strategies' Policy, Advocacy and Communications team for many years. Their respective subject matter expertise has allowed the creation of a unique research-to-action tool, bringing compelling evidence into the hands of advocates and policy-makers around the world.

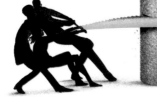

Friend

Member

🌐 Learn more at wecanprevent20.org

Working Together for Better Research
FCTC Article 5.2a Collaboration

COLLABORATORS

OUTPUT

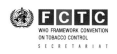

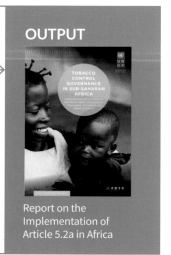

International observer to the FCTC and longtime global advocate of tobacco control	NGO from Kenya – longtime tobacco control proponent in Africa	The FCTC Secretariat helps Parties to enact the treaty's provisions	This UN organization is helping to make the strong link between tobacco control and development	Canadian academic institution

Report on the Implementation of Article 5.2a in Africa

These partners working closely with stakeholders across WHO FCTC parties, particularly tobacco control focal points and members of tobacco control intra-governmental coordinating mechanisms, to capture best practices (and worst nightmares) for multi-sectoral approaches to successful tobacco control.

REGULATING NOVEL PRODUCTS

📊 Problematic Ads

Appeals to youth

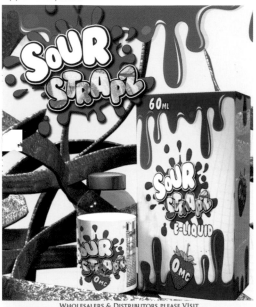

WHOLESALERS & DISTRIBUTORS PLEASE VISIT
WWW.FLAVORELIQUID.COM

Whom would this appeal to if not minors?

Appeals to ex-smokers

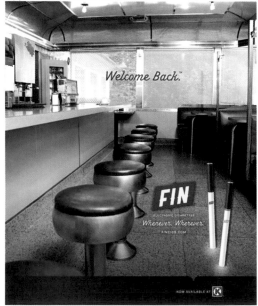

"Welcome Back" suggests an appeal to ex-smokers

E-cigarettes, the predominant type of electronic nicotine delivery system (ENDS), were originally designed to reduce smoking by replacing tobacco cigarettes, and there is limited but growing evidence that they are helping some smokers to transition away from combusted tobacco. The preponderance of available evidence suggests that using current-generation e-cigarettes is substantially less harmful than using tobacco cigarettes. However, there are lingering concerns about the harm from using e-cigarettes, particularly the uncertain long-term effects of nicotine use in the absence of combusted tobacco, and the interactions of heated e-liquid with sensitive lung tissue. There are also questions about whether e-cigarettes might pull ex-smokers back to using nicotine, and some argue that a causal "gateway effect" exists wherein youths begin to smoke tobacco cigarettes due to their exposure to e-cigarettes.

E-cigarettes present several regulatory challenges, and policymakers and governments continue to struggle with how to regulate them effectively. The most basic issue is whether these novel nicotine products should be given market access at all. At least 36 countries ban e-cigarette sales altogether, or permit device sales but ban the sale of nicotine e-liquid. This approach is under-standable for nations with very low smoking prevalence where introducing a new nicotine product might undermine tobacco control efforts. Most governments are trying a variety of other approaches to gatekeeping market access, ranging from permissive (e.g., similar to existing tobacco products) to more restrictive (e.g., requiring authorization from health authorities before entry into the market and on an ongoing basis) 📍.

Beyond market access, there are several other policies to consider. First, should existing tobacco cigarette regulations— e.g. excise taxes, public use bans, and market-ing restrictions —be applied to e-cigarettes,

and to what degree? Consider that many e-cigarette advertisements are blatantly directed at youth, recalling cigarette ads in the recent past 📊. Also, many countries have product safety regulations pertaining to e-liquid contents, child-safe packaging, nicotine quality and concentration, flavors, and other ingredients. Lastly, policymakers will need to consider what regulations should apply to "heat-not-burn" products that heat processed tobacco in a controlled fashion rather than combusting it 📊. They are likely to be more harmful than e-cigarettes because they contain tobacco, and the early evidence shows that they contain considerably higher levels of toxins than do e-cigarettes. There will not be much time to decide: heat-not-burn is already rapidly gaining market share in Japan, and has been introduced in more than 25 countries.

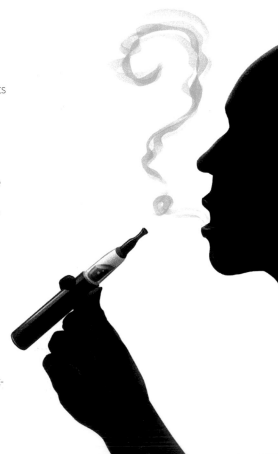

📍 Market Access Map

Uncertainty and controversy have contributed to wide variation in e-cigarette market access across the world

🌐 Explore more at ta6.org/regulating-novel-products

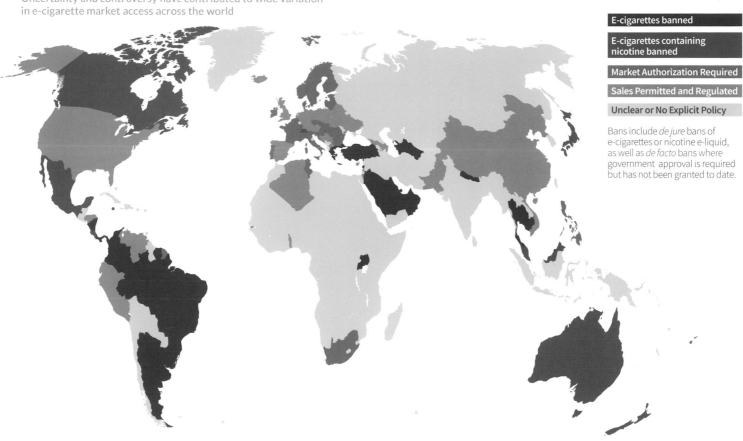

E-cigarettes banned

E-cigarettes containing nicotine banned

Market Authorization Required

Sales Permitted and Regulated

Unclear or No Explicit Policy

Bans include *de jure* bans of e-cigarettes or nicotine e-liquid, as well as *de facto* bans where government approval is required but has not been granted to date.

Extension of Tobacco Control Policies

Policy	Integration	Differentiation	Concerns
Smoking Bans	Extend existing bans to ENDS	ENDS allowed in public and private spaces	• Involuntary exposure to nicotine • Nuisance • Undermine cessation effect of smoking bans
Ad Bans	Extend all ad restrictions to ENDS	More permissive approach to placement and content of ENDS ads	• Youth and nonsmoker targeting • Sneaky smoking promotion
Warning Labels	Require warning label focused on toxicity	Focus on addiction, uncertainities, explosions	• Blurring line between harms of ENDS and greater harms of smoking
Taxes	Same taxes as other tobacco produts	Lower taxes than other tobacco products	• High enough price to reduce youth initiation • Price reflecting harm

📊 Slick retailing

Philip Morris is marketing their novel IQOS product in trendy stores with eager customer service representatives, resembling Apple Stores.

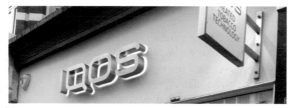

E-cigarette Device Types

E-cigarette and ENDS designs have evolved rapidly over the past decade

CIG-A-LIKE

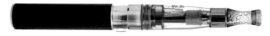

Cartridge that contains liquid nicotine and/or other ingredients

Sensor to detect when a smoker puffs

Heating mechanism to vaporize nicotine

Microprocessor to control heat and light

Battery

LED light

TANK STYLE

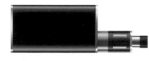

PERSONAL VAPORIZER

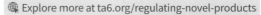

E-cigarettes are mainly either cig-a-like, tank systems, or personal vaporizer (PV).

Tank style and PV products are refillable with e-liquid.

Cig-a-likes can be disposable or re-useable.

CHAPTER 17
INDUSTRY STRATEGIES

When governments implement effective tobacco control policies, tobacco smoking declines. More quitting and less initiation of tobacco use contribute to greater individual and societal well-being. Successful tobacco control also hurts the financial health of tobacco companies. Consequently, tobacco companies act in their own interest, for example, by aggressively lobbying and litigating against government tobacco control policies, among other tactics.

In its zeal to promote tobacco use, the tobacco industry regularly perpetrates unethical, and often unlawful, interference with life-saving tobacco control policies. Although tobacco companies compete for market share, they often collude to counter government tobacco control efforts, or support front groups to do the job for them. Other strategies involve openly misrepresenting scientific evidence to confuse the public 📊.

Limiting this tobacco industry interference is possible. The WHO FCTC Article 5.3 guidelines identify specific limitations to the industry's involvement in policy-making, and outline strategies to limit the industry's participation and misconduct,

including paying close attention to the industry's actions. Industry monitoring programs are in place in many countries (including Brazil, South Africa, Sri Lanka, and the UK, among others). However, many governments do not report results from these monitoring efforts to the FCTC Secretariat as required by the treaty, nor is there sufficient effort yet to share this information among governments. Resources to address industry interference are also frequently lacking. International donors, such as the Bloomberg Philanthropies, have provided helpful funds for countries that lack capacity or resources to face multi-billion dollar companies in courts. Still, more stable funding mechanisms for legal support to governments are needed. In many places, directing funds from increases in tobacco taxes could help to bridge this gap.

UNDERMINING SCIENCE

Lower Visibility

LITIGATION

EVASION

LOBBYING AND HIJACKING LEGISLATIVE PROCESSES

Action

📊 Industry Interference

The tobacco industry deploys an array of strategies to undermine tobacco control efforts

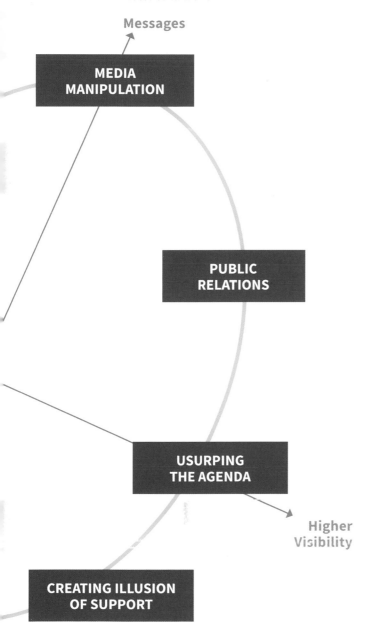

Messages

MEDIA MANIPULATION

PUBLIC RELATIONS

USURPING THE AGENDA

Higher Visibility

CREATING ILLUSION OF SUPPORT

UNDERMINING SCIENCE

The tobacco industry has long denied established scientific knowledge and popularized falsehoods, from deliberately clouding the links between smoking and lung cancer decades ago to misrepresenting the effects of plain packaging regulations now. In the US, they effectively utilized a small number of scientists to sow doubt about the hazards of smoking among policymakers and the public. The industry has promoted general mistrust toward science — a phenomenon that cripples global progress.

MEDIA MANIPULATION

The industry uses media to influence attitudes on a massive scale, often without disclosing funding, sponsorship, or authorship of content presented as objective "news". The industry secures content consistent with their interests by using advertising dollars to control media messages, by manufacturing information sources, or by ghostwriting pro-tobacco content. These messages underplay the benefits of proposed policies, exaggerate their costs, and overstate the industry's contribution to the economy and government revenue.

PUBLIC RELATIONS

Tobacco companies use philanthropy to link their public image with positive causes and build support among more credible groups, including local communities, NGOs, artistic/athletic organizations, academic institutions, or even governments and development agencies. When new tobacco control policies are on the agenda, the image of a good "corporate citizen" redirects attention away from the dire consequences of smoking.

USURPING THE AGENDA

The industry declares itself "part of the solution", but its ineffective voluntary measures cloud the regulatory space, often preventing or delaying implementation of effective policies. The industry previously launched campaigns to supposedly prevent youth smoking, which superficially appeared to warn against smoking, but were ultimately found to encourage kids to start smoking. The industry now proposes to "solve" challenges with illicit cigarettes via an industry-controlled tracking system, shifting power from governments to the industry. The industry also demands a voice in harm-reduction policy-making by claiming a commitment to producing less-harmful products. For example, Philip Morris International recently created a Foundation for a Smoke-Free World while continuing to actively promote their same lethal products.

CREATING ILLUSION OF SUPPORT

Front groups appear to serve a public cause but actually serve as the voice of the tobacco industry. These groups amplify industry messages by disguising the messenger, frequently giving policymakers the illusion of a broader coalition. The tobacco industry funds groups ranging from restaurant associations opposed to smoke-free laws, to large international think tanks against tax hikes. These groups repeatedly fail to disclose their funding and sponsorship, deceiving policymakers and the public about their true origin and intentions.

LOBBYING AND HIJACKING LEGISLATIVE PROCESSES

The industry uses political contributions and front groups to gain access to policymakers, and does not hesitate to provide ready-to-use legislative proposals. Governments determined to control tobacco use are being intimidated by messages misusing scientific evidence and misrepresenting effects of proposed regulations. In a particularly egregious example in 2017, the UK Serious Fraud Office opened an investigation into British American Tobacco involvement in bribing policymakers in at least four African countries: Burundi, Comoros, Kenya, and Rwanda.

EVASION

Once tobacco control legislation is passed, the industry often decides to deliberately circumvent or disobey the rules. One of the most damaging is the industry's involvement in the illicit cigarette trade, dodging tobacco taxes and supplying large quantities of their products through illegal channels.

🌐 Read more at ta6.org/illicit-trade

LITIGATION

Litigation has become one of the industry's deadliest weapons. The battles are fought at every level from domestic courts to international arbitration, where the vast legal resources of the large tobacco firms are commonly pitted against the often-limited legal resources of low- and medium-HDI countries. When the companies cannot directly bring a case, they use countries with lower public-policy standards to file formal disputes for them. The industry has been actively litigating tobacco control regulations in dozens of countries, while litigation threats "chill" similar measures in other countries, such as plain-packaging laws in New Zealand.

🌐 Read more at ta6.org/countering-the-industry

COUNTERING THE INDUSTRY

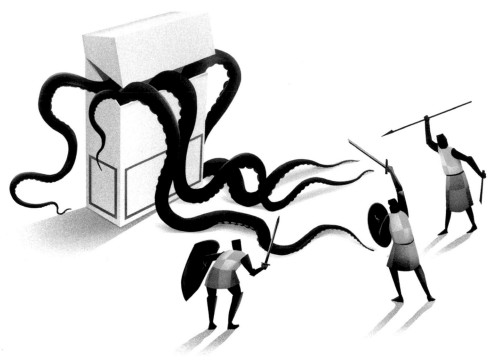

Tobacco control faces a most daunting foe in an enormous, highly-profitable, and politically well-connected tobacco industry driven to expand its customer base to maximize profits. However, there are proactive steps that the tobacco control community can take to counter the industry and maximize public health goals.

Preparation. One of the best strategies is to plan for the industry's inevitable pushback against any tobacco control effort that is likely to reduce their customer base — i.e., think before the implementation of an intervention. The tobacco industry typically employs the same set of strategies to fight against tobacco control efforts, no matter the time or place. For example, the industry continues to litigate against tobacco control policies in courts across the world, including claims that measures violate commitments to international economic agreements ♥. Anticipating that the industry would challenge their plain, standardized tobacco packaging initiative, Australia's health ministry worked in advance with its trade and foreign affairs counterparts to develop policy that would withstand scrutiny in trade dispute settlement, including in the World Trade Organization 📊.

Capacity. Effective tobacco control needs a variety of established professional skill sets, including economics, law, medicine, public health, social science, and communications to successfully execute policies and programs. For the countries lower on the Human Development Index, this will almost certainly mean some resource assistance, peer guidance, and targeted educational development from external supporters. The tobacco control community must escalate the engagement of appropriate professionals to outpace the industry's own hired experts.

Accountability. Governments must be accountable to their citizens, which includes ensuring overall societal well-being. Actively pursuing the straightforward obligations and recommendations of the WHO FCTC— including allocating sufficient resources to these efforts— will contribute to improved tobacco control, and therefore, greater societal well-being. The return on investment from tobacco control in lower health costs and increased productivity is enormous. Reliable and consistent measuring of progress can help to increase accountability.

Transparency. With near-constant pressure from the tobacco industry, governments must implement policies consistent with WHO FCTC Article 5.3 to make any interactions with the tobacco industry completely transparent— a crucial component of accountability. Moreover, the tobacco industry must have no place in shaping health policy or any policies that are likely to have health effects.

Multi-sectoral approach. As enshrined in WHO FCTC Article 5.2(a), for tobacco control to work more effectively, different sectors must work together. In the case of tobacco taxation, finance ministries must work with health counterparts to better understand how tax policy can maximize both revenues and health impacts. Health ministries are generally the natural tobacco control focal point, but they must understand their peer departments, and work to educate and empower them to vigorously promote tobacco control. Beyond government, civil society can help to pressure governments for better tobacco control and provide independent expertise, while the research sector can help to build tobacco control's evidence base.

♥ Tobacco Control and Litigation
Recent or current litigation against tobacco control efforts and/or litigation against the tobacco industry

🌐 Explore more at ta6.org/countering-the-industry

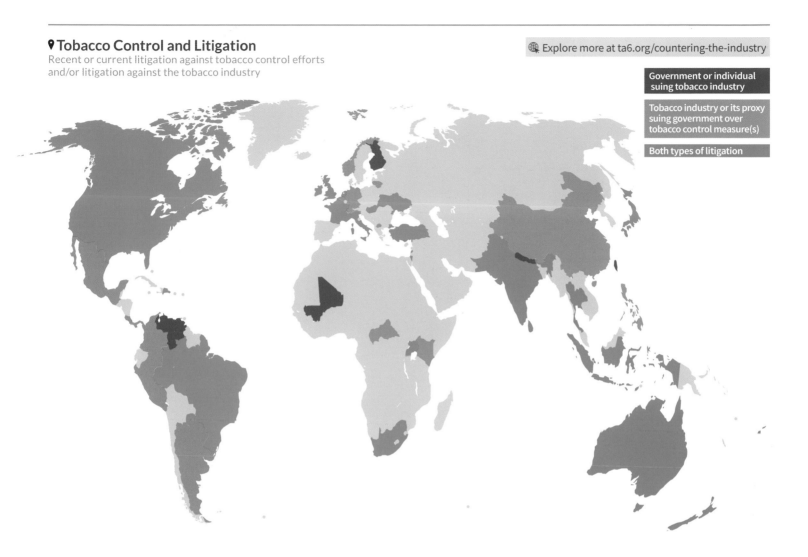

Government or individual suing tobacco industry

Tobacco industry or its proxy suing government over tobacco control measure(s)

Both types of litigation

The tobacco industry continues to aggressively litigate against tobacco control policies, but governments, the public health community and individuals have also been successfully using the courts to fight the tobacco industry's deadly ways.

▥ The World Trade Organization and Plain, Standardized Packaging
The WTO has become an important venue in which economic and health policies intersect

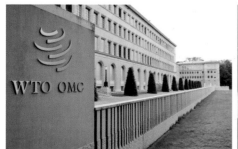

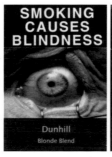

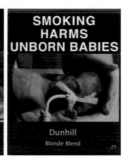

VENUE SHOPPING

The tobacco industry attempts to stop effective policies by any means necessary. Accordingly, they "shop" for the most favorable venue to do their bidding. Governments and tobacco control proponents need to understand these venues given the local context to neutralize the tobacco industry.

Venues include: legislatures; the courts (at all levels: municipal (e.g., local smoke-free ordinances), state/regional (e.g., taxation in some countries), and national (almost anything!)); and international bodies such as the World Trade Organization, trade agreements and bilateral investment treaties.

CHAPTER 19
OPTIMISM

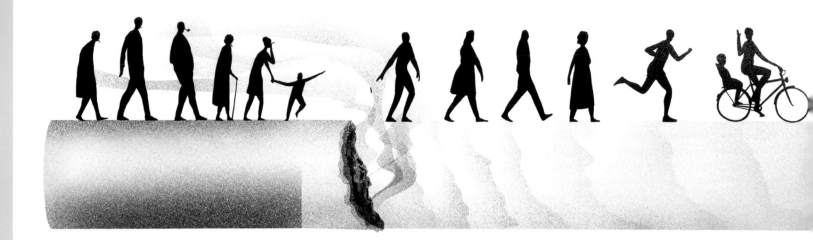

Global tobacco consumption is slowing. This is largely due to many countries implementing successful tobacco control programs. Slowly, the tobacco control community is "normalizing" its interventions. For example, a decade ago, just 10 countries had comprehensive smoke-free policies whereas today it is 55, with 23 more almost there. For those fortunate enough to live in smoke-free environments, it is thanks to these efforts that encountering smoking in a restaurant today feels so jarring. Once a society has adjusted to a smoke-free norm, it becomes difficult to understand why smoking was ever tolerated. But more work remains to be done.

Many tobacco control proponents aspire to a so-called "end game" for tobacco, and such visions vary considerably, from complete eradication of tobacco use to declines in prevalence to 5% or less. While it is important to aspire, we emphasize that vigorous implementation and enforcement of the proven strategies would undoubtedly drive tobacco prevalence down significantly and just as importantly keep low prevalence low. The largest obstacle in many countries remains a lack of will. Some government officials are still unwilling to follow through on commitments to the WHO FCTC, and more broadly, to commit sufficient

resources to promoting societal well-being through comprehensive tobacco control. Though there were small victories at the Seventh Conference of Parties of the WHO FCTC in late 2016, there were also disturbing signs of governments indifferent to tobacco control. Even worse, some official delegates promoted messages remarkably similar to those of the tobacco industry. These dynamics reinforce that the industry remains a powerful and ubiquitous force globally and must not be underestimated. However, an emerging global orientation toward preventing non-communicable diseases, and tobacco control's increasing place on the development agenda, are helping to challenge the industry's power.

There is considerable discussion in the public health community about the role of potentially less harmful tobacco products. This issue is complex. We implore readers to be open-minded but also skeptical, and to always turn to science – tobacco control must be grounded in facts. There may be no one-size-fits-all solution to this new challenge, but we must work together as a public health community, find or rigorously generate the necessary evidence, interpret it thoughtfully, and avoid dogmatism that serves to divide and potentially obfuscate important truths. While we must address new developments, we also cannot let them

distract from the key tasks at hand, particularly implementing evidence-based measures such as high excise taxes on cigarettes. New approaches to reducing tobacco-related disease will almost certainly work better in concert with proven measures to motivate quitting and discourage initiation. Moreover, there is no substitute for the weight of government action when it comes to implementing these proven measures.

As a modest start, we can set our sights on the established goal of a 30% relative reduction in prevalence by 2025 (from a 2010 baseline) with far more ambitious goals immediately thereafter. But governments must make a larger effort to implement these interventions and proponents working within government must raise their voices for change. And those outside of government, including civil society and researchers, must pressure governments to redouble their efforts, and provide assistance necessary to realizing these goals. We hope you will commit seriously to be part of this effort to save millions of lives from the scourge of tobacco use.

Please join us at www.tobaccoatlas.org, where you'll find additional exciting content and the most up-to-date data and developments as we work toward a tobacco-free future.

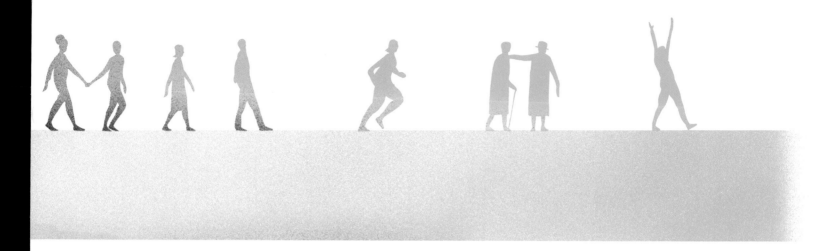

Tobacco Control Policy Implementation

Average performance across five major tobacco control policies:
smoke-free, warning labels, cessation, marketing bans and taxes

🌐 Explore more at la6.org/optimism

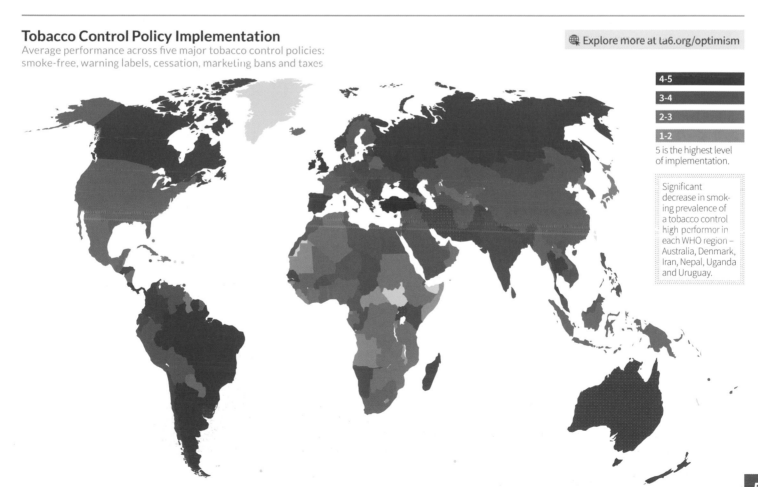

4-5	
3-4	
2-3	
1-2	

5 is the highest level
of implementation.

Significant
decrease in smok-
ing prevalence of
a tobacco control
high performer in
each WHO region –
Australia, Denmark,
Iran, Nepal, Uganda
and Uruguay.

INDEX